OFFICE OF POPULATION CENSUSES AND SURVEYS

TABULAR LIST OF THE CLASSIFICATION

OF

SURGICAL OPERATIONS AND PROCEDURES

FOURTH REVISION CONSOLIDATED VERSION 1990

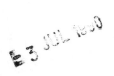
LONDON: HMSO

ISBN 0 11 691295 2

TABLE OF CONTENTS

INTRODUCTION

This is the consolidated version of the Office of Population Censuses and Surveys' Classification of Surgical Operations 4th revision, first issued in looseleaf form (OPCS,1987). It also incorporates updates to the classification issued in September 1987, December 1987, July 1988 and December 1989.

The classification has been devised as an instrument which will provide the best possible basis for accommodating current systems and future developments for data on surgical operations. As well as maintaining the planned objective, the classification also incorporates two further general aspects. It provides a definition of an operative procedure and outlines the concept of MAIN operation during an episode of care.

Historical Background

The earliest classification of surgical operations published in Britain was issued by the Medical Research Council in 1944. Using a simple 3-character code suitable for use with the punch card equipment available at the time, it identified 443 categories of operation. It is not known how extensively this preliminary classification was used in practice but its availability paved the way for a further scheme to be prepared by the then General Register Office in 1950. This took into account both the previous Medical Research Council version and a classification developed in 1949 for the United States Armed Forces, together with detailed specialist advice. This first GRO classification included 664 categories, again using a 3-character code; a 50 per cent increase on the MRC version. Subsequent additions were an index and two small series of 5-character codes for radiotherapy and anaesthetics. This classification was circulated widely for comment and used for trial purposes in a limited number of hospitals.

The generally favourable reaction to the 1950 classification prompted a first revision in a similar format. This was published in 1956, together with an index acknowledged at the time to be incomplete. The 1956 version contained slightly more categories (674), together with radiotherapeutic and anaesthetic supplements, and was reprinted in 1957. It was the first version used to routinely code records from the Hospital In-patient Enquiry but this process demonstrated some inadequacies not previously apparent. In consequence, a second revision was initiated in 1962 but not published until 1969; although a draft version was made available to some Regional Health Authorities in 1967 for use in coding Hospital Activity Analysis records. Whilst there was a further moderate increase in the number of 3-digit categories (to 731), the principal change was to provide optional fourth digit extensions in almost half the categories (353) and, as a result, to create 1183 definitive entries.

Whilst a reprint of the second revision, with some corrections, was issued in 1971, work started almost immediately on a third revision, eventually published in 1975. This revision was largely occasioned by a desire for comparability with the surgical operations section of a WHO International Classification of Procedures in Medicine being developed to coincide with the introduction of the 9th revision of the International Classification of Diseases. Only a very modest expansion, by three categories (to 734), was necessary at the 3-digit level for this purpose but the opportunity was taken for a considerable expansion in 4th digit sub-categories - increasing the definitive entries by one fifth (to 1426). Throughout the period from 1967 to 1985, there was an increasing availability of 4-digits but the central requirement for data remained at the level of the 3-digit code. Nevertheless, local users were encouraged to add and report such further 4th digit splits as were required. By 1985 some 2,000 individual codes had been notified in this way.

The increasing diversity of surgery carries the implication that any classification system for operations will rapidly lose its currency. Thus, not unexpectedly, the Steering Group on Health Services Information (chaired by Mrs E Korner) (SGHSI) in its first report in 1982 noted with concern (Para 5.40) that "the 1975 revision was by then several years out of date due to the continuous movement towards new operative techniques".

In consequence, the SGHSI recommended that, "as a matter of urgency, OPCS should provide operation codes which reflect current clinical practice and develop procedures for the frequent updating of the classification".

In response to this recommendation, one possible strategy was to adopt in Britain an existing classification from elsewhere. Three available English language versions were considered but were rejected for reasons other than the logistics and remoteness of source in relation to the dissemination of update information and to the establishment of any influence on its content. The already mentioned WHO International Classification of Procedures in Medicine, published in 1978, provides little more in the way of detail than the third revision of the OPCS classification and its structure precluded its use as a basis for national expansion. Consideration was also given to the possible adoption of either the Canadian classification of Diagnostic, Therapeutic and Surgical Procedures (published in 1978); or the United States' classification - included in the International Classification of Diseases, 9th revision: Clinical Modification (Vol 3) (published in 1979). Whilst these are more comprehensive than the WHO International Classification, they were found to be deficient on some aspects, particularly cardiac and vascular surgery. Finally, as none of these classifications was completely up to date, (although, subsequently, that from the United States was marginally updated in 1986), it seemed that the most appropriate course of action would be to issue a revised edition of the OPCS classification.

The revision process

Accordingly, in 1983 the process was begun to replace the outdated third revision, with the following general objectives:-

1. To identify and classify current surgical operations with particular reference to the incorporation of recent innovative techniques

2. To eliminate rarely performed operations but to include procedures not requiring the full operating theatre environment

3. To provide a flexible classification, responsive to less defined specialty boundaries and capable of future expansion

Initially, only limited modification was anticipated such that the existing framework could be used for the new fourth revision; but it soon became clear that more radical reconstruction was necessary. Thus, there is no similarity in the concept, approach or structure between the current revision and the revisions which precede it. However, the principle was maintained that the operation classification should not extend its role into functions properly within the scope of other classifications currently in use. Specifically, apart from a small number of justifiable exceptions, diagnostic parameters are excluded as these can be identified by reference to the International Classification of Diseases.

Classification or nomenclature?

Whereas some lists of diagnoses or surgical operations are designated as classifications, others are called nomenclatures; it is important to recognise that these two terms are neither synonymous nor interchangeable.

The difference in philosophy between a classification and a nomenclature was crystallised in 1965 by an expert group on Medical Terminology and Lexicography. This group was convened by the International Organisation for Medical Services (COIMS) under the then auspices of UNESCO and WHO. It defined a classification as:-

"a list of all the concepts belonging to a well defined group (eg of diagnoses etc) compiled in accordance with criteria enabling them to be arranged systematically, and permitting the establishment of a hierarchy based on the natural or logical relationship between them".

Furthermore, the group explicitly drew attention to the fundamental difference from a <u>nomenclature</u> by continuing the definition:-

"a classification should not be confused with a nomenclature. Whereas the latter is simply a list of names, a classification is an attempt to establish a logical hierarchy between the concepts themselves. The name of a concept may change without affecting the place of the concept in the classification".

The disparity was further emphasised by the definition of a <u>nomenclature</u> as:-

"a systematic list, in one or several languages, of all or as many names as possible of members of a clearly defined conceptual or linguistic family, usually without accompanying definitions. Thus the names of all plants constitute a botanical nomenclature, and so with animals, tumours, diseases, etc".

Thus, in short, a nomenclature of diseases or surgical operations is a list of names, whilst a classification is a list of concepts. Nevertheless, the distinction tends to be blurred as there is obvious advantage in listing a nomenclature in a logical order; and encompassing all acceptable terms in a classification. However, the difference is not merely theoretical, for, through usage, it has also become functional. Long standing classifications, such as the International Classification of Diseases, have been designed explicitly for the compilation of statistics, especially those of a routine nature. In contrast, traditional nomenclatures, such as the Nomenclature of Disease published by the Royal College of Physicians (until 1960), served to identify acceptable terminology.

Arising out of these substantive differences in function, each category in a classification is invariably assigned a code number in fixed format, allocated in a way that will facilitate aggregation of individual categories for statistical purposes. Such an assignment is irrelevant for an entry in a 'pure' nomenclature. However, there is a further function for which a classification is frequently used, but for which it is not ideally designed; namely to provide an index to enable records to be retrieved for research purposes. Since classifications, of diagnoses or operations, by definition frequently encompass a number of different entities within a single concept, it is inappropriate to judge them on the basis of a singular ability - the absence of which may well be highlighted within the research context (namely that of uniquely identifying 'new' diseases or operations) - outside of the definition of their expressed function.

Equally, such diverse requirements are not going to be completely satisfied by a nomenclature. Those nomenclatures which have been developed more recently incorporate sophisticated features to allow highly specific indexing. For example, the Standard Nomenclature of Medicine (SNOMED), compiled by the College of American Pathologists, has the ability to identify any diagnostic or operation term for research purposes. The SNOMED system lists a code for each of six possible component parameters (eg topography, morphology or type of procedure) which might be associated with any term; each code incorporates a prefix indicating the parameter. Unique identification of any term is achieved by 'stringing' these component codes together and a satisfactory 'string' can be constructed even if the complete term is not previously 'known' to the system.

'Strings' generated in this way are usually complex and frequently not of fixed length. Whilst these characteristics are not incompatible with an index constructed for record access, they do create severe problems for routine analysis. When it is further considered that derived combination codes may fail to fit within an established hierarchy of concepts, a situation is created which virtually negates the use of such systems, in their present form, as a basis for the compilation of routine statistics.

Of course this does not preclude any attempt to develop computer or other routines to assign every possible 'string' to an appropriate category in a statistical classification; provided that the nomenclature encompasses all the concepts required by that classification. However, in addition to the basic problems stemming from essential difference in their expressed function, assignment difficulties will be exacerbated by a fact inherent in the current situation. A revised classification will inevitably introduce innovations outside the scope of current nomenclatures - just as a reissue of a nomenclature would be likely to include new terms for which provision would be lacking in an existing classification.

It is neither the function of this classification to establish a standard nomenclature of surgical operations nor even to suggest that one should be used. Rather, it is designed to accommodate and appropriately assign as many as possible of the terminologies that are likely to be recorded.

The structure of the classification

In basic structure, this Tabular List comprises 23 anatomically based chapters, most of which relate to the whole or part of a system of the body and each is designated alphabetically; eg Chapter A covers the nervous system and Chapter K the heart. Strict anatomical allocation of operations has infused a readily understandable logic into the classification - essential, given the increased blurring of specialty boundaries. For example, Chapter A now includes operations usually associated with orthopaedic surgery - eg neurolysis; with vascular surgery - eg sympathectomy; and with gastroenterological surgery - eg vagotomy; as well as those traditionally the province of neurosurgery.

The alphabetic character for each chapter forms the leading digit of the 3 and 4-digit codes within it. Previous revisions used all-numeric codes and the innovation of an alphanumeric format has increased the potential capacity of the revision from 999 to 2277 3-digit categories (not 2574, since - to avoid confusion - I, O and U are not used). As issued, a total of 1178 (subsequently updated to 1183) 3-digit categories were defined; separately identifying over 4000 specified 4-digit sub-categories. Each 3-digit category is presented in similar format (Figure 1) and usually includes the provision of two sub-categories designated as 'other specified' and 'unspecified'.

Figure 1

Q32	**Operations on fimbria**
Q32.1	Excision of fimbria
Q32.2	Burying of fimbria in wall of uterus
Q32.3	Excision of hydatid of morgagni
Q32.8	Other specified
Q32.9	Unspecified

As it is not yet established surgical practice to use only English terms when recording operations, a mixture of English and Classical descriptions is used at the 4-digit level. However, only English terms are used in 3-digit titles so that these categories are expressed and arranged in such a way that their content is consistent, clear and unequivocal, despite some apparently tortuous wording to the uninitiated. Also, in line with previous advice, the use of eponyms is discouraged and such terms are excluded from the Tabular List.

Whatever detailed provision is made at the 4-digit level, the 3-digit categories form the backbone of the classification and their ordering and designation merit particular emphasis. In keeping with the general anatomical structure of the classification, each chapter is sub-divided into separate 'organ' sections. The sub-divisions in Chapter M (the urinary tract), for example, are the kidney; ureter; bladder; etc.

Within each section, procedures have been generally sequenced in a way which reflects their comparative significance in resource use terms. Although they are often implicitly allocated to groups labelled as 'major', 'intermediate' or 'minor', there are, at present, no acceptably defined criteria whereby operations can be classed in this way. In this classification, a more pragmatic approach is taken whereby, within each organ section, the procedures listed are presented broadly in descending order of complexity. Thus, operations for removal of an organ usually precede those for its repair, which in turn come before lesser procedures such as aspiration or manipulation. As an important part of this process, particular attention has been paid to the categorisation of less invasive techniques such as endoscopic surgery. These have been specifically segregated from open operations on the same organ and, in turn, therapeutic procedures of this nature are usually separated from diagnostic ones which use a similar approach.

In line with previous practice, this tabular list also incorporates a number of inclusion terms, exclusion terms and notes, which will assist in the correct assignment of an appropriate code.

Innovations

Space in this introduction does not permit the inclusion of a comprehensive survey of the detailed additions or changes that will be found by thorough inspection of the revision but a small selection of the more obvious innovations is shown in Figure 2. Attention is drawn, for example, to the incorporation of microsurgery, the use of lasers and extracorporeal lithotripsy; as well as the identification of important techniques in prosthetic joint and arterial surgery.

Figure 2

A03.3	Stereotactic ablation of tissue of globus pallidus
B14.1	Global parathyroidectomy and transposition of parathyroid tissue
D24.1	Implantation of intracochlear prosthesis
E34.1	Microtherapeutic endoscopic extirpation of lesion of larynx using laser
F11.2	Augmentation of alveolar ridge using autobone graft
G03.2	Partial oesophagectomy and interposition of mictovascularly attached jejunum
H30.1	Radiological reduction of intussusception of colon using barium enema
J10.1	Percutaneous transluminal embolisation of hepatic artery
J16.2	Extracorporeal assistance to liver
J43.1	Endoscopic retrograde cholangiopancreatography and biopsy of lesion of ampulla of vater
K49.2	Percutaneous transluminal balloon angioplasty of multiple coronary arteries
L48.1	Emergency replacement of aneurysmal common iliac artery by anastomosis of aorta to common iliac artery
M09.2	Endoscopic electrohydraulic shock wave fragmentation of calculus of kidney
R05.3	Percutaneous sampling of chorionic villus
S05.1	Microscopically controlled excision of lesion of skin of head or neck using fresh tissue technique
S48.2	Insertion of skin expander into subcutaneous tissue of breast
T45.1	Image controlled percutaneous drainage of subphrenic abscess
T76.1	Microvascular free tissue transfer of flap of muscle
T86.2	Sampling of axillary lymph nodes
V41.1	Posterior attachment of correctional instrument to spine
X05.2	Implantation of kineplastic prosthesis for limb

Previous editions of the classification included a number of conventions by which certain (sometimes less familiar) terms were invested with special meanings in order to enhance the clarity of specification of some categories. For example, the term <u>lesion</u> of an organ is again used to describe any localised pathology, whether neoplastic, infective or degenerative; its <u>extirpation</u> covers either its excision or its destruction by whatever means.

This practice has been extended in the reissued revision; for example the term <u>intubation</u> is generally restricted to situations where a tube is introduced into an organ and then withdrawn; whereas, when the tube is left in-situ, the term <u>insertion of tube</u> is normally used. For operations involving a <u>prosthesis</u>, a special terminology is used to cover the various associated procedures (Figure 3).

Figure 3

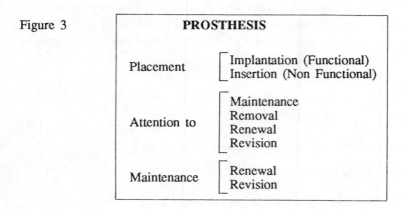

Single procedure analysis and Multiple coding

When a series of operations is recorded, it is traditional, as with diagnostic information, to select the first mentioned for routine analysis.

With diagnostic information, the International Classification of diseases recommends criteria for the selection of the MAIN condition for single cause analysis. Accordingly, in conjunction with this operation classification, it is logical to propose that <u>the operation to be selected for single procedure analysis from records of episodes of hospital care should be the MAIN operation or procedure carried out during the relevant episodes; the choice of which, wherever possible, should be exercised by the responsible person,</u>

Hitherto, the first named operation may have been the MAIN one performed; alternatively, it could have been the first carried out chronologically, thus allowing the opportunity for inconsistencies in statistical analysis. With identification of the MAIN operation and its assignment to the 'first coded' position, many of these inconsistencies would be eliminated. However, unlike the practice for diagnostic information, it has not proved possible to promulgate rules or procedures to assist coders in the selection of the MAIN operation in instances when it is not identified by the surgeon.

Sometimes multiple operations are carried out simultaneously. Hitherto, the methods adopted for their classification have lacked an obvious rationale. Some combinations have been encompassed within a single category, whilst others, with a seemingly similar relationship, have required to be coded separately. Both methods are again adopted in the present revision but are used more logically, with, in general, operations carried out in combination requiring the use of multiple codes; particularly when more than one organ is involved. The general rules provided above for the selection of the main operation when more than one is performed have been used to give specific guidance as to which operation should take precedence in cases where traditionally paired operations, such as 'tonsillectomy' and 'adenoidectomy', are separated. Thus, 'vagotomy' is deemed to be the main operation when carried out together with 'gastrojejunostomy'.

A single entry in the classification is still used on occasion to cover multiple procedures on the same organ, for example:-

J33.1   Open removal of calculus from bile duct and drainage of bile duct

This mechanism is also used to reduce what would otherwise be a multiplicity of codes. For example, a single code cannot cover the various options for radical or extended mastectomy but one series of 4th digit categories within:-

B27   Total excision of breast

does include both the mastectomy and various degrees of local extension into the chest wall; leaving the use of a further code (eg T86.2) to identify the extent of lymph node removal.

Improved arrangements for the classification of multiple procedures carried out simultaneously should not be confused with another innovation - the facility to code additional detail using a wide range of supplementary codes. Two complete chapters of the revision are allocated for this purpose, as is one unique fourth digit (.0).

Chapter Y provides 'Methods of Operation' codes which are intended for the incorporation of otherwise unclassifiable detail in a far wider range of procedures. For example, Y08 covers different types of laser procedure and can thus identify the use of this form of treatment whenever associated with a particular operation. It is not intended that the additional codes derived from this chapter should 'stand alone'. Consequently, provision has been made in Chapter X ('Miscellaneous Operations') for a series of codes designed to precede codes in Chapter Y where more precise preceding codes cannot be determined or are not available.

Chapter Z gives a series of site codes which may provide a useful facility for the identification of intra-organ anatomical detail. For example, Z15 delineates the various quadrants of the breast. However, the use of these codes is essential in the appropriate anatomical classification of orthopaedic surgery.

The further facility of this nature, particularly appropriate to orthopaedic surgery, is the provision of codes such as:-

W57.0 Conversion from previous excision arthroplasty of joint

which allow the incorporation of information about previous procedures which have to be 'dismantled' as part of the current operation, with obvious resource implications.

It is, of course, intended that these purely descriptive codes will be excluded from any statistical count of operations performed. It is to comply with this requirement that they are identifiable by a unique prefix or suffix.

Definition of an operative procedure

Operative procedures are those carried out on patients undergoing treatment

- for the prevention, diagnosis, care or relief of disease
- for the correction of deformity or deficit, including those performed for cosmetic reasons
- associated with pregnancy, childbirth or contraceptive or procreative management

and will <u>normally</u> involve:-

1. performance in an operating theatre

2. by a surgeon (in a training or career post)

3. aseptic measures

4. anaesthesia (eg general, spinal or epidural anaesthesia or infiltration with local anaesthetic) more elaborate than basal sedation administered on the ward or self administered inhalation

5. techniques including incision, excision or destruction of tissue, plastic repair or reconstruction, interventional radiology, puncture beyond the skin and subcutaneous tissue, cautery, diathermy, cryosurgery, photocoagulation, endoscopy, dilation, removal of foreign bodies, catheterisation or forced manipulation.

This 4th revision does include categories in Chapter Y (Y80 onwards) which may be used to code certain activities which fall outside of the above definitions.

Scope of the Classification

The 4th revision of the classification is intended to be used in conjunction with other available classifications such as:-

1. The 9th revision of the ICD

2. A classification of surgical specialties

3. Methods of classification of urgency of admission eg emergency or elective

Thus, it was neither intended that the classification, or groups from it, should be used as a substitute for these other classifications nor, in general, that elements from these should be included in the category descriptions. Some minor exceptions to this general rule are unavoidable.

Radical operations

Radical operations are usually neither listed nor tabulated as such in the classification.

The term 'radical' can imply an operation on more than one site - eg removal of an organ and its associated lymph nodes.

It can allude to the extent of the operation within the site(s) - eg modified radical mastectomy.

Therefore, it is essential to ensure, by recourse to the originator if necessary, that the operations statement provides a detailed definition of 'radical' in terms which facilitate the assignment of the correct codes(s).

Incomplete or failed operations or procedures

These should be coded to the stage reached at the abandonment of the operation or procedure.

The <u>intention</u> should not be coded.

Index to the Classification

A copy of the index to this classification is available on floppy disk from:

> The WHO Centre
> Office of Population Censuses and Surveys
> Segensworth Road
> Titchfield
> Fareham
> Hants
> PO15 5RR

The index will be re-issued annually or as required.

Abbreviations

Four specific abbreviations are used in this volume; their meaning is as follows:-

hfq	However further qualified
nec	Not elsewhere classified
nfq	Not further qualified
noc	Not otherwise classifiable

References

Office of Population Censuses and Surveys. Classification of Surgical Operations and Procedures, Fourth revision, 1987. London, OPCS, 1987.

Medical Research Council. A Provisional Classification of Diseases and Injuries for use in Compiling Morbidity Statistics. Special Report Series No 248. London, HMSO, 1944.

General Register Office. Draft Code of Surgical Operations. London, GRO, 1950.

General Register Office. Code of Surgical Operations, 1956. London, HMSO, 1956.

General Register Office. Classification of Surgical Operations, Second Revision, 1969. London, GRO, 1969.

Office of Population Censuses and Surveys. Classification of Surgical Operations, Third Revision, 1975. London, OPCS, 1975.

World Health Organisation. Manual of the International Statistical Classification of Diseases, Injuries, and Causes of Death, 9th Revision, 1975. Geneva, WHO, 1977.

Steering Group on Health Services Information. Chairman: Mrs E Korner. First Report to the Secretary of State. London, HMSO, 1982.

World Health Organisation. International Classification of Procedures in Medicine. Geneva, WHO, 1978.

Nosology Reference Centre, Statistics Canada. Canadian Classification of Diagnostic, Therapeutic, and Surgical Procedures. Ottawa, Statistics Canada, 1978.

United States Department of Health and Human Services. The International Classification of Diseases, 9th Revision: Clinical Modification, Vol 3 Procedures, Second Edition, 1980. PH5 80-1260. Washington, US Government Publishing Office, 1980.

Council for International Organisations of Medical Sciences. Medical Terminology and Lexicography. Basel, Karger, 1966.

Royal College of Physicians of London. The Nomenclature of Disease, 8th Edition. London, HMSO, 1960.

College of American Pathologists. SNOMED: Systematized Nomenclature of Medicine. Skokie, Illinois, CAP, 1977

ACKNOWLEDGEMENTS

The Office of Population Censuses and Surveys wishes to thank the members of the Steering Group set up to oversee this revision of the Classification of Surgical Operations and Procedures. Particular tribute must be paid to the willing help given by members of the Information Division of the Common Services Agency Scottish Health Service, especially Dr J Webb.

The following organisations were consulted during the development of the classification:-

Association of Anaesthetists of Great Britain and Ireland
Association of British Clinical Neurophysiologists
Association of British Neurologists
Association of Health Care Information and Medical Records Officers
Back Pain Association Ltd
British Association of Audiological Physicians
British Association of Dermatologists
British Association of Otolaryngologists
British Association of Paediatric Surgeons
British Association of Plastic Surgeons
British Association of Urological Surgeons
British Cardiac Society
British Medical Laser Association
British Orthopaedic Association
British Society of Gastroenterology
British Society of Rheumatology
British Thoracic Society
British Transplantation Society
Casualty Surgeons Association
Faculty of Anaesthetists, Royal College of Surgeons of England
Faculty of Dental Surgery, Royal College of Surgeons of England
Intensive Care Society
Intractable Pain Association of Great Britain and Ireland
JCHST SAC Accident and Emergency
JCHST SAC Cardiothoracic Surgery
JCHST SAC General Surgery
JCHST SAC Neurological Surgery
JCHST SAC Ophthalmology
JCHST SAC Orthopaedic Surgery
JCHST SAC Otolaryngology
JCHST SAC Paediatric Surgery
JCHST SAC Plastic Surgery
JCHST SAC Urology
Medico-Social Research Board
Royal College of General Practitioners
Royal College of Obstetricians and Gynaecologists
Royal College of Physicians of Edinburgh
Royal College of Physicians of London
Royal College of Physicians and Surgeons of Glasgow
Royal College of Radiologists
Royal College of Surgeons of Edinburgh
Royal College of Surgeons of England
Society of British Neurological Surgeons
Society of Chiropodists
Society of Thoracic and Cardiovascular Surgeons of Great Britain and Ireland
Vascular Surgical Society of Great Britain and Ireland

OPCS is indebted to these organisations and their representatives for the invaluable contributions they have made. The revision would not have been possible without this help. Furthermore, the advice and comments received from health authorities and a large number of interested individuals have enhanced the scope of the revision and are also gratefully acknowledged.

TABULAR LIST OF THREE DIGIT CATEGORIES

A. NERVOUS SYSTEM

Tissue of brain (A01-A10)

A01 Major excision of tissue of brain
A02 Excision of lesion of tissue of brain
A03 Stereotactic ablation of tissue of brain
A04 Open biopsy of lesion of tissue of brain
A05 Drainage of lesion of tissue of brain
A07 Other open operations on tissue of brain
A08 Other biopsy of lesion of tissue of brain
A09 Neurostimulation of brain
A10 Other operations on tissue of brain

Ventricle of brain and subarachnoid space (A12-A22)

A12 Creation of connection from ventricle of brain
A13 Attention to component of connection from ventricle of brain
A14 Other operations on connection from ventricle of brain
A16 Other open operations on ventricle of brain
A17 Therapeutic endoscopic operations on ventricle of brain
A18 Diagnostic endoscopic examination of ventricle of brain
A20 Other operations on ventricle of brain
A22 Operations on subarachnoid space of brain

Cranial nerves (A24-A36)

A24 Graft to cranial nerve
A25 Intracranial transection of cranial nerve
A26 Other intracranial destruction of cranial nerve
A27 Extracranial extirpation of vagus nerve (x)
A28 Extracranial extirpation of other cranial nerve
A29 Excision of lesion of cranial nerve
A30 Repair of cranial nerve
A31 Intracranial stereotactic release of cranial nerve
A32 Other decompression of cranial nerve
A33 Neurostimulation of cranial nerve
A34 Exploration of cranial nerve
A36 Other operations on cranial nerve

Meninges of brain (A38-A42)

A38 Extirpation of lesion of meninges of brain
A39 Repair of dura
A40 Drainage of extradural space
A41 Drainage of subdural space
A42 Other operations on meninges of brain

Spinal cord and other contents of spinal canal (A44-A57)

A44 Partial extirpation of spinal cord
A45 Other open operations on spinal cord
A47 Other destruction of spinal cord
A48 Other operations on spinal cord
A49 Repair of spina bifida
A51 Other operations on meninges of spinal cord
A52 Therapeutic epidural injection
A53 Drainage of spinal canal
A54 Therapeutic spinal puncture
A55 Diagnostic spinal puncture
A57 Operations on spinal nerve root

Peripheral nerves (A59-A73)

A59 Excision of peripheral nerve
A60 Destruction of peripheral nerve
A61 Extirpation of lesion of peripheral nerve
A62 Microsurgical repair of peripheral nerve
A63 Other graft to peripheral nerve
A64 Other repair of peripheral nerve
A65 Release of entrapment of peripheral nerve at wrist
A66 Release of entrapment of peripheral nerve at ankle
A67 Release of entrapment of peripheral nerve at other site
A68 Other release of peripheral nerve
A69 Revision of release of peripheral nerve
A70 Neurostimulation of peripheral nerve
A73 Other operations on peripheral nerve

Other parts of nervous system (A75-A84)

A75 Excision of cervical sympathetic nerve
A76 Chemical destruction of sympathetic nerve
A77 Cryotherapy to sympathetic nerve
A78 Radiofrequency controlled thermal destruction of sympathetic nerve
A79 Other destruction of sympathetic nerve
A81 Other operations on sympathetic nerve
A83 Electroconvulsive therapy
A84 Neurophysiological operations

B. ENDOCRINE SYSTEM AND BREAST

Pituitary and pineal glands (B01-B06)

B01 Excision of pituitary gland
B02 Destruction of pituitary gland
B04 Other operations on pituitary gland
B06 Operations on pineal gland

Thyroid and parathyroid glands (B08-B16)

B08 Excision of thyroid gland
B09 Operations on aberrant thyroid tissue
B10 Operations on thyroglossal tissue
B12 Other operations on thyroid gland
B14 Excision of parathyroid gland
B16 Other operations on parathyroid gland

Other endocrine glands (B18-B25)

B18 Excision of thymus gland
B20 Other operations on thymus gland
B22 Excision of adrenal gland
B23 Operations on aberrant adrenal tissue
B25 Other operations on adrenal gland

Breast (B27-B37)

B27 Total excision of breast
B28 Other excision of breast
B29 Reconstruction of breast
B30 Prosthesis for breast
B31 Other plastic operations on breast
B32 Biopsy of breast
B33 Incision of breast
B34 Operations on duct of breast
B35 Operations on nipple
B36 Other operations on breast
B37 Other operations on breast

4

C. EYE

Orbit (C01-C08)

C01 Excision of eye
C02 Extirpation of lesion of orbit
C03 Insertion of prosthesis of eye
C04 Attention to prosthesis of eye
C05 Plastic repair of orbit
C06 Incision of orbit
C08 Other operations on orbit

Eyebrow and eyelid (C10-C22)

C10 Operations on eyebrow
C11 Operations on canthus
C12 Extirpation of lesion of eyelid
C13 Excision of redundant skin of eyelid
C14 Reconstruction of eyelid
C15 Correction of deformity of eyelid
C16 Other plastic repair of eyelid
C17 Other repair of eyelid
C18 Correction of ptosis of eyelid
C19 Incision of eyelid
C20 Protective suture of eyelid
C22 Other operations on eyelid

Lacrimal apparatus (C24-C29)

C24 Operations on lacrimal gland
C25 Connection between lacrimal apparatus and nose
C26 Other operations on lacrimal sac
C27 Operations on nasolacrimal duct
C29 Other operations on lacrimal apparatus

Muscles of eye (C31-C37)

C31 Combined operations on muscles of eye
C32 Recession of muscle of eye
C33 Resection of muscle of eye
C34 Partial division of tendon of muscle of eye
C35 Other adjustment to muscle of eye
C37 Other operations on muscle of eye

Conjunctiva and cornea (C39-C51)

C39 Extirpation of lesion of conjunctiva
C40 Repair of conjunctiva
C41 Incision of conjunctiva
C43 Other operations on conjunctiva
C45 Extirpation of lesion of cornea
C46 Plastic operations on cornea
C47 Closure of cornea
C48 Removal of foreign body from cornea
C49 Incision of cornea
C51 Other operations on cornea

Sclera and iris (C53-C64)

C53 Extirpation of lesion of sclera
C54 Buckling operations for attachment of retina
C55 Incision of sclera
C57 Other operations on sclera
C59 Excision of iris
C60 Filtering operations on iris
C61 Other operations on trabecular meshwork of eye
C62 Incision of iris
C64 Other operations on iris

Anterior chamber of eye and lens (C66-C77)

C66 Extirpation of ciliary body
C67 Other operations on ciliary body
C69 Other operations on anterior chamber of eye
C71 Extracapsular extraction of lens
C72 Intracapsular extraction of lens
C73 Incision of capsule of lens
C74 Other extraction of lens
C75 Prosthesis of lens
C77 Other operations on lens

Retina and other parts of eye (C79-C86)

C79 Operations on vitreous body
C81 Photocoagulation of retina for detachment
C82 Destruction of lesion of retina
C84 Other operations on retina
C86 Other operations on eye

D. EAR

External ear and external auditory canal (D01-D08)

D01 Excision of external ear
D02 Extirpation of lesion of external ear
D03 Plastic operations on external ear
D04 Drainage of external ear
D06 Other operations on external ear
D07 Clearance of external auditory canal
D08 Other operations on external auditory canal

Mastoid and middle ear (D10-D20)

D10 Exenteration of mastoid air cells
D12 Other operations on mastoid
D14 Repair of eardrum
D15 Drainage of middle ear
D16 Reconstruction of ossicular chain
D17 Other operations on ossicle of ear
D19 Extirpation of lesion of middle ear
D20 Other operations on middle ear

Inner ear and eustachian canal (D22-D28)

D22 Operations on eustachian canal
D24 Operations on cochlea
D26 Operations on vestibular apparatus
D28 Other operations on ear

E. RESPIRATORY TRACT

Nose (E01-E10)

E01   Excision of nose
E02   Plastic operations on nose
E03   Operations on septum of nose
E04   Operations on turbinate of nose
E05   Surgical arrest of bleeding from internal nose
E06   Packing of cavity of nose
E08   Other operations on internal nose
E09   Operations on external nose
E10   Other operations on nose

Nasal sinuses (E12-E17)

E12   Operations on maxillary antrum using sublabial approach
E13   Other operations on maxillary antrum
E14   Operations on frontal sinus
E15   Operations on sphenoid sinus
E17   Operations on unspecified nasal sinus

Pharynx (E19-E27)

E19   Excision of pharynx
E20   Operations on adenoid
E21   Repair of pharynx
E23   Other open operations on pharynx
E24   Therapeutic endoscopic operations on pharynx
E25   Diagnostic endoscopic examination of pharynx
E27   Other operations on pharynx

Larynx (E29-E38)

E29   Excision of larynx
E30   Open extirpation of lesion of larynx
E31   Reconstruction of larynx
E33   Other open operations on larynx
E34   Microtherapeutic endoscopic operations on larynx
E35   Other therapeutic endoscopic operations on larynx
E36   Diagnostic endoscopic examination of larynx
E38   Other operations on larynx

Trachea and bronchus (E39-E52)

E39   Partial excision of trachea
E40   Plastic operations on trachea
E41   Open placement of prosthesis in trachea
E42   Exteriorisation of trachea
E43   Other open operations on trachea
E44   Open operations on carina
E46   Partial extirpation of bronchus
E47   Other open operations on bronchus
E48   Therapeutic fibreoptic endoscopic operations on lower respiratory tract
E49   Diagnostic fibreoptic endoscopic examination of lower respiratory tract
E50   Therapeutic endoscopic operations on lower respiratory tract using bronchoscope
E51   Diagnostic endoscopic examination of lower respiratory tract using rigid bronchoscope
E52   Other operations on bronchus

Lung and mediastinum (E53-E63)

E53 Transplantation of lung
E54 Excision of lung
E55 Open extirpation of lesion of lung
E57 Other open operations on lung
E59 Other operations on lung
E61 Open operations on mediastinum
E62 Therapeutic endoscopic operations on mediastinum
E63 Diagnostic endoscopic examination of mediastinum

F. MOUTH

Lip (F01-F06)

F01 Partial excision of lip
F02 Extirpation of lesion of lip
F03 Correction of deformity of lip
F04 Other reconstruction of lip
F05 Other repair of lip
F06 Other operations on lip

Tooth and gingiva (F08-F20)

F08 Implantation of tooth
F09 Surgical removal of tooth
F10 Simple extraction of tooth
F11 Preprosthetic oral surgery
F12 Surgery on apex of tooth
F13 Restoration of tooth
F14 Orthodontic operations
F16 Other operations on tooth
F18 Excision of dental lesion of jaw
F20 Operations on gingiva

Tongue and palate (F22-F32)

F22 Excision of tongue
F23 Extirpation of lesion of tongue
F24 Incision of tongue
F26 Other operations on tongue
F28 Extirpation of lesion of palate
F29 Correction of deformity of palate
F30 Other repair of palate
F32 Other operations on palate

Tonsil and other parts of mouth (F34-F42)

F34 Excision of tonsil
F36 Other operations on tonsil
F38 Extirpation of lesion of other part of mouth
F39 Reconstruction of other part of mouth
F40 Other repair of other part of mouth
F42 Other operations on mouth

Salivary apparatus (F44-F58)

F44 Excision of salivary gland
F45 Extirpation of lesion of salivary gland
F46 Incision of salivary gland
F48 Other operations on salivary gland
F50 Transposition of salivary duct
F51 Open extraction of calculus from salivary duct
F52 Ligation of salivary duct
F53 Other open operations on salivary duct
F55 Dilation of salivary duct
F56 Manipulative removal of calculus from salivary duct
F58 Other operations on salivary duct

G. UPPER DIGESTIVE TRACT

Oesophagus including hiatus hernia (G01-G25)

G01 Excision of oesophagus and stomach
G02 Total excision of oesophagus
G03 Partial excision of oesophagus
G04 Open extirpation of lesion of oesophagus
G05 Bypass of oesophagus
G06 Attention to connection of oesophagus
G07 Repair of oesophagus
G08 Artificial opening into oesophagus
G09 Incision of oesophagus
G10 Open operations on varices of oesophagus
G11 Open placement of prosthesis in oesophagus
G13 Other open operations on oesophagus
G14 Fibreoptic endoscopic extirpation of lesion of oesophagus
G15 Other therapeutic fibreoptic endoscopic operations on oesophagus
G16 Diagnostic fibreoptic endoscopic examination of oesophagus
G17 Endoscopic extirpation of lesion of oesophagus using rigid oesophagoscope
G18 Other therapeutic endoscopic operations on oesophagus using rigid oesophagoscope
G19 Diagnostic endoscopic examination of oesophagus using rigid oesophagoscope
G21 Other operations on oesophagus
G23 Repair of diaphragmatic hernia
G24 Antireflux operations
G25 Revision of antireflux operations

Stomach pylorus and general upper gastrointestinal tract endoscopy (G27-G48)

G27 Total excision of stomach
G28 Partial excision of stomach
G29 Open extirpation of lesion of stomach
G30 Plastic operations on stomach
G31 Connection of stomach to duodenum
G32 Connection of stomach to transposed jejunum
G33 Other connection of stomach to jejunum
G34 Artificial opening into stomach
G35 Operations on ulcer of stomach
G36 Other repair of stomach
G38 Other open operations on stomach
G40 Incision of pylorus
G41 Other operations on pylorus
G43 Fibreoptic endoscopic extirpation of lesion of upper gastrointestinal tract
G44 Other fibreoptic therapeutic endoscopic operations on upper gastrointestinal tract
G45 Diagnostic fibreoptic endoscopic examination of upper gastrointestinal tract
G47 Intubation of stomach
G48 Other operations on stomach

Duodenum (G49-G57)

G49 Excision of duodenum
G50 Open extirpation of lesion of duodenum
G51 Bypass of duodenum
G52 Operations on ulcer of duodenum
G53 Other open operations on duodenum
G54 Therapeutic endoscopic operations on duodenum
G55 Diagnostic endoscopic examination of duodenum
G57 Other operations on duodenum

Jejunum (G58-G67)

G58 Excision of jejunum
G59 Extirpation of lesion of jejunum
G60 Artificial opening into jejunum
G61 Bypass of jejunum
G62 Open endoscopic operations on jejunum
G63 Other open operations on jejunum
G64 Therapeutic endoscopic operations on jejunum
G65 Diagnostic endoscopic examination of jejunum
G67 Other operations on jejunum

Ileum (G69-G82)

G69 Excision of ileum
G70 Open extirpation of lesion of ileum
G71 Bypass of ileum
G72 Other connection of ileum
G73 Attention to connection of ileum
G74 Creation of artificial opening into ileum
G75 Attention to artificial opening into ileum
G76 Intraabdominal manipulation of ileum
G78 Other open operations on ileum
G79 Therapeutic endoscopic operations on ileum
G80 Diagnostic endoscopic examination of ileum
G82 Other operations on ileum

H. LOWER DIGESTIVE TRACT

Appendix (H01-H03)

H01 Emergency excision of appendix
H02 Other excision of appendix
H03 Other operations on appendix

Colon (H04-H30)

H04 Total excision of colon and rectum
H05 Total excision of colon
H06 Extended excision of right hemicolon
H07 Other excision of right hemicolon
H08 Excision of transverse colon
H09 Excision of left hemicolon
H10 Excision of sigmoid colon
H11 Other excision of colon
H12 Extirpation of lesion of colon
H13 Bypass of colon
H14 Exteriorisation of caecum
H15 Other exteriorisation of colon
H16 Incision of colon
H17 Intraabdominal manipulation of colon
H18 Open endoscopic operations on colon
H19 Other open operations on colon
H20 Endoscopic extirpation of lesion of colon

H21	Other therapeutic endoscopic operations on colon
H22	Diagnostic endoscopic examination of colon
H23	Endoscopic extirpation of lesion of lower bowel using fibreoptic sigmoidoscope
H24	Other therapeutic endoscopic operations on lower bowel using fibreoptic sigmoidoscope
H25	Diagnostic endoscopic examination of lower bowel using fibreoptic sigmoidoscope
H26	Endoscopic extirpation of lesion of sigmoid colon using rigid sigmoidoscope
H27	Other therapeutic endoscopic operations on sigmoid colon using rigid sigmoidoscope
H28	Diagnostic endoscopic examination of sigmoid colon using rigid sigmoidoscope
H30	Other operations on colon

Rectum (H32-H46)

H33	Excision of rectum
H34	Open extirpation of lesion of rectum
H35	Fixation of rectum for prolapse
H36	Other abdominal operations for prolapse of rectum
H40	Operations on rectum through anal sphincter
H41	Other operations on rectum through anus
H42	Perineal operations for prolapse of rectum
H44	Manipulation of rectum
H46	Other operations on rectum

Anus and perianal region (H47-H62)

H47	Excision of anus
H48	Excision of lesion of anus
H49	Destruction of lesion of anus
H50	Repair of anus
H51	Excision of haemorrhoid
H52	Destruction of haemorrhoid
H53	Other operations on haemorrhoid
H54	Dilation of anal sphincter
H55	Other operations on perianal region
H56	Other operations on anus
H58	Drainage through perineal region
H59	Excision of pilonidal sinus
H60	Other operations on pilonidal sinus
H62	Other operations on bowel

J. OTHER ABDOMINAL ORGANS - PRINCIPALLY DIGESTIVE

Liver (J01-J16)

J01	Transplantation of liver
J02	Partial excision of liver
J03	Extirpation of lesion of liver
J04	Repair of liver
J05	Incision of liver
J07	Other open operations on liver
J08	Therapeutic endoscopic operations on liver using laparoscope
J09	Diagnostic endoscopic examination of liver using laparoscope
J10	Transluminal operations on blood vessel of liver
J12	Other therapeutic percutaneous operations on liver
J13	Diagnostic percutaneous operations on liver
J14	Other puncture of liver
J16	Other operations on liver

Gall bladder (J18-J26)

J18　Excision of gall bladder
J19　Connection of gall bladder
J20　Repair of gall bladder
J21　Incision of gall bladder
J23　Other open operations on gall bladder
J24　Therapeutic percutaneous operations on gall bladder
J25　Diagnostic percutaneous operations on gall bladder
J26　Other operations on gall bladder

Bile duct (J27-J52)

J27　Excision of bile duct
J28　Extirpation of lesion of bile duct
J29　Connection of hepatic duct
J30　Connection of common bile duct
J31　Open introduction of prosthesis into bile duct
J32　Repair of bile duct
J33　Incision of bile duct
J34　Plastic repair of sphincter of Oddi using duodenal approach
J35　Incision of sphincter of Oddi using duodenal approach
J36　Other operations on ampulla of Vater using duodenal approach
J37　Other open operations on bile duct
J38　Endoscopic incision of sphincter of Oddi
J39　Other therapeutic endoscopic operations on ampulla of Vater
J40　Endoscopic retrograde placement of prosthesis in bile duct
J41　Other therapeutic endoscopic retrograde operations on bile duct
J42　Therapeutic endoscopic retrograde operations on pancreatic duct
J43　Diagnostic endoscopic retrograde examination of bile duct and pancreatic duct
J44　Diagnostic endoscopic retrograde examination of bile duct
J45　Diagnostic endoscopic retrograde examination of pancreatic duct
J46　Therapeutic percutaneous attention to connection of bile duct
J47　Therapeutic percutaneous insertion of prosthesis into bile duct
J48　Other therapeutic percutaneous operations on bile duct
J49　Therapeutic operations on bile duct along T tube track
J50　Percutaneous examination of bile duct
J52　Other operations on bile duct

Pancreas (J54-J67)

J54　Transplantation of pancreas
J55　Total excision of pancreas
J56　Excision of head of pancreas
J57　Other partial excision of pancreas
J58　Extirpation of lesion of pancreas
J59　Connection of pancreatic duct
J60　Other open operations on pancreatic duct
J61　Open drainage of lesion of pancreas
J62　Incision of pancreas
J63　Open examination of pancreas
J65　Other open operations on pancreas
J66　Therapeutic percutaneous operations on pancreas
J67　Diagnostic percutaneous operations on pancreas

Spleen (J69-J72)

J69　Total excision of spleen
J70　Other excision of spleen
J72　Other operations on spleen

K. HEART

Wall septum and chambers of heart (K01-K23)

K01   Transplantation of heart and lung
K02   Other transplantation of heart
K04   Correction of tetralogy of fallot
K05   Atrial inversion operations for transposition of great vessels
K06   Other correction of transposition of great vessels
K07   Correction of total anomalous pulmonary venous connection
K09   Closure of defect of atrioventricular septum
K10   Closure of defect of interatrial septum
K11   Closure of defect of interventricular septum
K12   Closure of defect of unspecified septum of heart
K14   Other open operations on septum of heart
K15   Closed operations on septum of heart
K16   Therapeutic transluminal operations on septum of heart
K18   Creation of valved cardiac conduit
K19   Creation of other cardiac conduit
K20   Refashioning of atrium
K22   Other operations on wall of atrium
K23   Other operations of wall of heart

Valves of heart and adjacent structures (K25-K38)

K25   Plastic repair of mitral valve
K26   Plastic repair of aortic valve
K27   Plastic repair of tricuspid valve
K28   Plastic repair of pulmonary valve
K29   Plastic repair of unspecified valve of heart
K30   Revision of plastic repair of valve of heart
K31   Open incision of valve of heart
K32   Closed incision of valve of heart
K34   Other open operations on valve of heart
K35   Therapeutic transluminal operations on valve of heart
K37   Removal of obstruction from structure adjacent to valve of heart
K38   Other operations on structure adjacent to valve of heart

Coronary artery (K40-K51)

K40   Saphenous vein graft replacement of coronary artery
K41   Other autograft replacement of coronary artery
K42   Allograft replacement of coronary artery
K43   Prosthetic replacement of coronary artery
K44   Other replacement of coronary artery
K45   Connection of thoracic artery to coronary artery
K46   Other bypass of coronary artery
K47   Repair of coronary artery
K48   Other open operations on coronary artery
K49   Transluminal balloon angioplasty of coronary artery
K50   Other therapeutic transluminal operations on coronary artery
K51   Diagnostic transluminal operations on coronary artery

Other parts of heart and pericardium (K52-K71)

K52   Open operations on conducting system of heart
K53   Other incision of heart
K55   Other open operations on heart
K56   Transluminal heart assist operations
K57   Other therapeutic transluminal operations on heart
K58   Diagnostic transluminal operations on heart
K60   Cardiac pacemaker system introduced through vein
K61   Other cardiac pacemaker system
K63   Contrast radiology of heart
K65   Catheterisation of heart
K66   Other operations on heart

K67   Excision of pericardium
K68   Drainage of pericardium
K69   Incision of pericardium
K71   Other operations on pericardium

L. ARTERIES AND VEINS

Great vessels and pulmonary artery (L01-L13)

L01   Open operations for combined abnormality of great vessels
L02   Open correction of patent ductus arteriosus
L03   Transluminal operations on abnormality of great vessel
L05   Creation of shunt to pulmonary artery from aorta using interposition tube prosthesis
L06   Other connection to pulmonary artery from aorta
L07   Creation of shunt to pulmonary artery from subclavian artery using interposition tube prosthesis
L08   Other connection to pulmonary artery from subclavian artery
L09   Other connection to pulmonary artery
L10   Repair of pulmonary artery
L12   Other open operations on pulmonary artery
L13   Transluminal operations on pulmonary artery

Aorta (L16-L26)

L16   Extraanatomic bypass of aorta
L18   Emergency replacement of aneurysmal segment of aorta
L19   Other replacement of aneurysmal segment of aorta
L20   Other emergency bypass of segment of aorta
L21   Other bypass of segment of aorta
L22   Attention to prosthesis of aorta
L23   Plastic repair of aorta
L25   Other open operations on aorta
L26   Transluminal operations on aorta

Carotid cerebral and subclavian arteries (L29-L39)

L29   Reconstruction of carotid artery
L30   Other open operations on carotid artery
L31   Transluminal operations on carotid artery
L33   Operations on aneurysm of cerebral artery
L34   Other open operations on cerebral artery
L35   Transluminal operations on cerebral artery
L37   Reconstruction of subclavian artery
L38   Other open operations on subclavian artery
L39   Transluminal operations on subclavian artery

Abdominal branches of aorta (L41-L47)

L41   Reconstruction of renal artery
L42   Other open operations on renal artery
L43   Transluminal operations on renal artery
L45   Reconstruction of other visceral branch of abdominal aorta
L46   Other open operations on other visceral branch of abdominal aorta
L47   Transluminal operations on other visceral branch of abdominal aorta

Iliac and femoral arteries (L48-L63)

L48   Emergency replacement of aneurysmal iliac artery
L49   Other replacement of aneurysmal iliac artery
L50   Other emergency bypass of iliac artery
L51   Other bypass of iliac artery
L52   Reconstruction of iliac artery
L53   Other open operations on iliac artery
L54   Transluminal operations on iliac artery
L56   Emergency replacement of aneurysmal femoral artery
L57   Other replacement of aneurysmal femoral artery
L58   Other emergency bypass of femoral artery
L59   Other bypass of femoral artery
L60   Reconstruction of femoral artery
L62   Other open operations on femoral artery
L63   Transluminal operations on femoral artery

Other arteries (L65-L72)

L65   Revision of reconstruction of artery
L67   Excision of other artery
L68   Repair of other artery
L70   Other open operations on other artery
L71   Therapeutic transluminal operations on other artery
L72   Diagnostic transluminal operations on other artery

Veins and other blood vessels (L74-L97)

L74   Arteriovenous shunt
L75   Other arteriovenous operations
L77   Connection of vena cava or branch of vena cava
L79   Other operations on vena cava
L81   Other bypass operations on vein
L82   Repair of valve of vein
L83   Other operations for venous insufficiency
L85   Ligation of varicose vein of leg
L86   Injection into varicose vein of leg
L87   Other operations on varicose vein of leg
L90   Open removal of thrombus from vein
L91   Other vein related operations
L93   Other open operations on vein
L94   Therapeutic transluminal operations on vein
L95   Diagnostic transluminal operations on vein
L97   Other operations on blood vessel

M. URINARY

Kidney (M01-M16)

M01   Transplantation of kidney
M02   Total excision of kidney
M03   Partial excision of kidney
M04   Open extirpation of lesion of kidney
M05   Open repair of kidney
M06   Incision of kidney
M08   Other open operations on kidney
M09   Therapeutic endoscopic operations on calculus of kidney
M10   Other therapeutic endoscopic operations on kidney
M11   Diagnostic endoscopic examination of kidney
M13   Percutaneous puncture of kidney
M14   Extracorporeal fragmentation of calculus of kidney
M15   Operations on kidney along nephrostomy tube track
M16   Other operations on kidney

Ureter (M18-M32)

M18   Excision of ureter
M19   Urinary diversion
M20   Replantation of ureter
M21   Other connection of ureter
M22   Repair of ureter
M23   Incision of ureter
M25   Other open operations on ureter
M26   Therapeutic nephroscopic operations on ureter
M27   Therapeutic ureteroscopic operations on ureter
M28   Other endoscopic removal of calculus from ureter
M29   Other therapeutic endoscopic operations on ureter
M30   Diagnostic endoscopic examination of ureter
M31   Extracorporeal fragmentation of calculus of ureter
M32   Operations on ureteric orifice

Bladder (M34-M49)

M34   Total excision of bladder
M35   Partial excision of bladder
M36   Enlargement of bladder
M37   Other repair of bladder
M38   Open drainage of bladder
M39   Other open operations on contents of bladder
M41   Other open operations on bladder
M42   Endoscopic extirpation of lesion of bladder
M43   Endoscopic operations to increase capacity of bladder
M44   Other therapeutic endoscopic operations on bladder
M45   Diagnostic endoscopic examination of bladder
M47   Urethral catheterisation of bladder
M49   Other operations on bladder

Outlet of bladder and prostate (M51-M70)

M51   Combined abdominal and vaginal operations to support outlet of female bladder
M52   Abdominal operations to support outlet of female bladder
M53   Vaginal operations to support outlet of female bladder
M55   Other open operations on outlet of female bladder
M56   Therapeutic endoscopic operations on outlet of female bladder
M58   Other operations on outlet of female bladder
M61   Open excision of prostate
M62   Other open operations on prostate
M64   Other open operations on outlet of male bladder
M65   Endoscopic resection of outlet of male bladder
M66   Other therapeutic endoscopic operations on outlet of male bladder
M67   Other therapeutic endoscopic operations on prostate
M70   Other operations on outlet of male bladder

Urethra and other parts of urinary tract (M72-M83)

M72   Excision of urethra
M73   Repair of urethra
M75   Other open operations on urethra
M76   Therapeutic endoscopic operations on urethra
M77   Diagnostic endoscopic examination of urethra
M79   Other operations on urethra
M81   Operations on urethral orifice
M83   Other operations on urinary tract

N. MALE GENITAL ORGANS

Scrotum and testis (N01-N13)

N01   Extirpation of scrotum
N03   Other operations on scrotum
N05   Bilateral excision of testes
N06   Other excision of testis
N07   Extirpation of lesion of testis
N08   Bilateral placement of testes in scrotum
N09   Other placement of testis in scrotum
N10   Prosthesis of testis
N11   Operations on hydrocele sac
N13   Other operations on testis

Spermatic cord and male perineum (N15-N24)

N15   Operations on epididymis
N17   Excision of vas deferens
N18   Repair of spermatic cord
N19   Operations on varicocele
N20   Other operations on spermatic cord
N22   Operations on seminal vesicle
N24   Operations on male perineum

Penis and other male genital organs (N26-N34)

N26   Amputation of penis
N27   Extirpation of lesion of penis
N28   Plastic operations on penis
N29   Prosthesis of penis
N30   Operations on prepuce
N32   Other operations on penis
N34   Other operations on male genital tract

P. LOWER FEMALE GENITAL TRACT

Vulva and female perineum (P01-P13)

P01   Operations on clitoris
P03   Operations on Bartholin gland
P05   Excision of vulva
P06   Extirpation of lesion of vulva
P07   Repair of vulva
P09   Other operations on vulva
P11   Extirpation of lesion of female perineum
P13   Other operations on female perineum

Vagina (P14-P31)

P14   Incision of introitus of vagina
P15   Other operations on introitus of vagina
P17   Excision of vagina
P18   Other obliteration of vagina
P19   Excision of band of vagina
P20   Extirpation of lesion of vagina
P21   Plastic operations on vagina
P22   Repair of prolapse of vagina and amputation of cervix uteri
P23   Other repair of prolapse of vagina
P24   Repair of vault of vagina
P25   Other repair of vagina
P26   Introduction of supporting pessary into vagina
P27   Exploration of vagina
P29   Other operations on vagina
P31   Operations on pouch of Douglas

Q. UPPER FEMALE GENITAL TRACT

Uterus (Q01-Q20)

Q01   Excision of cervix uteri
Q02   Destruction of lesion of cervix uteri
Q03   Biopsy of cervix uteri
Q05   Other operations on cervix uteri
Q07   Abdominal excision of uterus
Q08   Vaginal excision of uterus
Q09   Other open operations on uterus
Q10   Curettage of uterus
Q11   Other evacuation of contents of uterus
Q12   Intrauterine contraceptive device
Q13   Introduction of gamete into uterine cavity
Q14   Introduction of abortifacient into uterine cavity
Q15   Introduction of other substance into uterine cavity
Q16   Other vaginal operations on uterus
Q17   Therapeutic endoscopic operations on uterus
Q18   Diagnostic endoscopic examination of uterus
Q20   Other operations on uterus

Fallopian tube (Q22-Q41)

Q22   Bilateral excision of adnexa of uterus
Q23   Unilateral excision of adnexa of uterus
Q24   Other excision of adnexa of uterus
Q25   Partial excision of fallopian tube
Q26   Placement of prosthesis in fallopian tube
Q27   Open bilateral occlusion of fallopian tubes
Q28   Other open occlusion of fallopian tube
Q29   Open reversal of female sterilisation
Q30   Other repair of fallopian tube
Q31   Incision of fallopian tube
Q32   Operations on fimbria
Q34   Other open operations on fallopian tube
Q35   Endoscopic bilateral occlusion of fallopian tubes
Q36   Other endoscopic occlusion of fallopian tube
Q37   Endoscopic reversal of female sterilisation
Q38   Other therapeutic endoscopic operations on fallopian tube
Q39   Diagnostic endoscopic examination of fallopian tube
Q41   Other operations on fallopian tube

Ovary and broad ligament (Q43-Q56)

Q43   Partial excision of ovary
Q44   Open destruction of lesion of ovary
Q45   Repair of ovary
Q47   Other open operations on ovary
Q48   Oocyte recovery
Q49   Therapeutic endoscopic operations on ovary
Q50   Diagnostic endoscopic examination of ovary
Q52   Operations on broad ligament of uterus
Q54   Operations on other ligament of uterus
Q55   Other examination of female genital tract
Q56   Other operations on female genital tract

R. FEMALE GENITAL TRACT ASSOCIATED WITH PREGNANCY CHILDBIRTH AND PUERPERIUM

Fetus and gravid uterus (R01-R12)

R01 Therapeutic endoscopic operations on fetus
R02 Diagnostic endoscopic examination of fetus
R03 Selective destruction of fetus
R04 Therapeutic percutaneous operations on fetus
R05 Diagnostic percutaneous examination of fetus
R10 Other operations on amniotic cavity
R12 Operations on gravid uterus

Induction and delivery (R14-R27)

R14 Surgical induction of labour
R15 Other induction of labour
R17 Elective caesarean delivery
R18 Other caesarean delivery
R19 Breech extraction delivery
R20 Other breech delivery
R21 Forceps cephalic delivery
R22 Vacuum delivery
R23 Cephalic vaginal delivery with abnormal presentation of head at delivery without instrument
R24 Normal delivery
R25 Other methods of delivery
R27 Other operations to facilitate delivery

Other obstetric (R28-R34)

R28 Instrumental removal of products of conception from delivered uterus
R29 Manual removal of products of conception from delivered uterus
R30 Other operations on delivered uterus
R32 Immediate repair of obstetric laceration
R34 Other obstetric operations

S. SKIN

Skin or subcutaneous tissue (S01-S62)

S01 Plastic excision of skin of head or neck
S02 Plastic excision of skin of abdominal wall
S03 Plastic excision of skin of other site
S04 Other excision of skin
S05 Microscopically controlled excision of lesion of skin
S06 Other excision of lesion of skin
S08 Curettage of lesion of skin
S09 Photodestruction of lesion of skin
S10 Other destruction of lesion of skin of head or neck
S11 Other destruction of lesion of skin of other site
S13 Punch biopsy of skin
S14 Shave biopsy of skin
S15 Other biopsy of skin
S17 Distant flap of skin and muscle
S18 Distant flap of skin and fascia
S19 Distant pedicle flap of skin
S20 Other distant flap of skin
S21 Hair bearing flap of skin
S22 Sensory flap of skin
S23 Flap operations to relax contracture of skin
S24 Local flap of skin and muscle
S25 Local flap of skin and fascia
S26 Local subcutaneous pedicle flap of skin
S27 Other local flap of skin
S28 Flap of mucosa

S30	Other operations on flap of skin to head or neck
S31	Other operations on flap of skin to other site
S33	Hair bearing graft of skin to scalp
S34	Hair bearing graft of skin to other site
S35	Split autograft of skin
S36	Other autograft of skin
S37	Other graft of skin
S38	Graft of mucosa
S39	Graft of other tissue to skin
S41	Suture of skin of head or neck
S42	Suture of skin of other site
S43	Removal of repair material from skin
S44	Removal of other inorganic substance from skin
S45	Removal of other substance from skin
S47	Opening of skin
S48	Insertion of skin expander into subcutaneous tissue
S49	Attention to skin expander in subcutaneous tissue
S50	Introduction of other inert substance into subcutaneous tissue
S51	Introduction of destructive substance into subcutaneous tissue
S52	Introduction of therapeutic substance into subcutaneous tissue
S53	Introduction of substance into skin
S54	Exploration of burnt skin of head or neck
S55	Exploration of burnt skin of other site
S56	Exploration of other skin of head or neck
S57	Exploration of other skin of other site
S60	Other operations on skin
S62	Other operations on subcutaneous tissue

Nail (S64-S70)

S64	Extirpation of nail bed
S66	Other operations on nail bed
S68	Excision of nail
S70	Other operations on nail

T. SOFT TISSUE

Chest wall pleura and diaphragm (T01-T17)

T01	Partial excision of chest wall
T02	Reconstruction of chest wall
T03	Opening of chest
T05	Other operations on chest wall
T07	Open excision of pleura
T08	Open drainage of pleural cavity
T09	Other open operations on pleura
T10	Therapeutic endoscopic operations on pleura
T11	Diagnostic endoscopic examination of pleura
T12	Puncture of pleura
T13	Introduction of substance into pleural cavity
T14	Other operations on pleura
T15	Repair of rupture of diaphragm
T16	Other repair of diaphragm
T17	Other operations on diaphragm

Abdominal wall (T19-T31)

T19 Simple excision of inguinal hernial sac
T20 Primary repair of inguinal hernia
T21 Repair of recurrent inguinal hernia
T22 Primary repair of femoral hernia
T23 Repair of recurrent femoral hernia
T24 Repair of umbilical hernia
T25 Primary repair of incisional hernia
T26 Repair of recurrent incisional hernia
T27 Repair of other hernia of abdominal wall
T28 Other repair of anterior abdominal wall
T29 Operations on umbilicus
T30 Opening of abdomen
T31 Other operations on anterior abdominal wall

Peritoneum (T33-T48)

T33 Open extirpation of lesion of peritoneum
T34 Open drainage of peritoneum
T36 Operations on omentum
T37 Operations on mesentery of small intestine
T38 Operations on mesentery of colon
T39 Operations on posterior peritoneum
T41 Other open operations on peritoneum
T42 Therapeutic endoscopic operations on peritoneum
T43 Diagnostic endoscopic examination of peritoneum
T45 Image controlled operations on abdominal cavity
T46 Other drainage of peritoneal cavity
T48 Other operations on peritoneum

Fascia ganglion and bursa (T50-T62)

T50 Transplantation of fascia
T51 Excision of fascia of abdomen
T52 Excision of other fascia
T53 Extirpation of lesion of fascia
T54 Division of fascia
T55 Release of fascia
T57 Other operations on fascia
T59 Excision of ganglion
T60 Reexcision of ganglion
T62 Operations on bursa

Tendon (T64-T74)

T64 Transposition of tendon
T65 Excision of tendon
T67 Primary repair of tendon
T68 Secondary repair of tendon
T69 Freeing of tendon
T70 Adjustment to length of tendon
T71 Excision of sheath of tendon
T72 Other operations on sheath of tendon
T74 Other operations on tendon

Muscle (T76-T83)

T76 Transplantation of muscle
T77 Excision of muscle
T79 Repair of muscle
T80 Release of contracture of muscle
T81 Biopsy of muscle
T83 Other operations on muscle

Lymphatic tissue (T85-T96)

T85   Block dissection of lymph nodes
T86   Sampling of lymph nodes
T87   Excision or biopsy of lymph node
T88   Drainage of lesion of lymph node
T89   Operations on lymphatic duct
T90   Contrast radiology of lymphatic tissue
T92   Other operations on lymphatic tissue
T94   Operations on bronchial cleft
T96   Other operations on soft tissue

V. BONES AND JOINTS OF SKULL AND SPINE

Bones and joints of cranium, face and jaw (V01-V21)

V01   Plastic repair of cranium
V03   Opening of cranium
V05   Other operations on cranium
V07   Excision of bone of face
V08   Reduction of fracture of maxilla
V09   Reduction of fracture of other bone of face
V10   Division of bone of face
V11   Fixation of bone of face
V13   Other operations on bone of face
V14   Excision of mandible
V15   Reduction of fracture of mandible
V16   Division of mandible
V17   Fixation of mandible
V19   Other operations on mandible
V20   Reconstruction of temporomandibular joint
V21   Other operations on temporomandibular joint

Bones and joints of spine (V22-V54)

V22   Primary decompression operations on cervical spine
V23   Revisional decompression operations on cervical spine
V24   Decompression operations on thoracic spine
V25   Primary decompression operations on lumbar spine
V26   Revisional decompression operations on lumbar spine
V27   Decompression operations on unspecified spine
V29   Primary excision of cervical intervertebral disc
V30   Revisional excision of cervical intervertebral disc
V31   Primary excision of thoracic intervertebral disc
V32   Revisional excision of thoracic intervertebral disc
V33   Primary excision of lumbar intervertebral disc
V34   Revisional excision of lumbar intervertebral disc
V35   Excision of unspecified intervertebral disc
V37   Primary fusion of joint of cervical spine
V38   Primary fusion of other joint of spine
V39   Revisional fusion of joint of spine
V41   Instrumental correction of deformity of spine
V42   Other correction of deformity of spine
V43   Extirpation of lesion of spine
V44   Decompression of fracture of spine
V45   Other reduction of fracture of spine
V46   Fixation of fracture of spine
V47   Biopsy of spine
V48   Denervation of spinal facet joint of vertebra
V49   Exploration of spine
V50   Manipulation of spine
V52   Other operations on intervertebral disc
V54   Other operations on spine

W. OTHER BONES AND JOINTS

Complex reconstruction of hand and foot (W01-W04)

W01   Complex reconstruction of thumb
W02   Other complex reconstruction of hand
W03   Complex reconstruction of forefoot
W04   Complex reconstruction of hindfoot

Bone (W06-W36)

W05   Prosthetic replacement of bone
W06   Total excision of bone
W07   Excision of ectopic bone
W08   Other excision of bone
W09   Extirpation of lesion of bone
W10   Open surgical fracture of bone
W11   Other surgical fracture of bone
W12   Angulation periarticular division of bone
W13   Other periarticular division of bone
W14   Diaphyseal division of bone
W15   Division of bone of foot
W16   Other division of bone
W17   Other reconstruction of bone
W18   Drainage of bone
W19   Primary open reduction of fracture of bone and intramedullary fixation
W20   Primary open reduction of fracture of bone and extramedullary fixation
W21   Primary open reduction of intraarticular fracture of bone
W22   Other primary open reduction of fracture of bone
W23   Secondary open reduction of fracture of bone
W24   Closed reduction of fracture of bone and internal fixation
W25   Closed reduction of fracture of bone and external fixation
W26   Other closed reduction of fracture of bone
W27   Fixation of epiphysis
W28   Other internal fixation of bone
W29   Skeletal traction of bone
W30   Other external fixation of bone
W31   Other autograft of bone
W32   Other graft of bone
W33   Other open operations on bone
W34   Graft of bone marrow
W35   Therapeutic puncture of bone
W36   Diagnostic puncture of bone

Joint (W37-W92)

W37   Total prosthetic replacement of hip joint using cement
W38   Total prosthetic replacement of hip joint not using cement
W39   Other total prosthetic replacement of hip joint
W40   Total prosthetic replacement of knee joint using cement
W41   Total prosthetic replacement of knee joint not using cement
W42   Other total prosthetic replacement of knee joint
W43   Total prosthetic replacement of other joint using cement
W44   Total prosthetic replacement of other joint not using cement
W45   Other total prosthetic replacement of other joint
W46   Prosthetic replacement of head of femur using cement
W47   Prosthetic replacement of head of femur not using cement
W48   Other prosthetic replacement of head of femur
W49   Prosthetic replacement of head of humerus using cement
W50   Prosthetic replacement of head of humerus not using cement
W51   Other prosthetic replacement of head of humerus
W52   Prosthetic replacement of articulation of other bone using cement
W53   Prosthetic replacement of articulation of other bone not using cement
W54   Other prosthetic replacement of articulation of other bone
W55   Prosthetic interposition reconstruction of joint
W56   Other interposition reconstruction of joint

W57 Excision reconstruction of joint
W58 Other reconstruction of joint
W59 Fusion of joint of toe
W60 Fusion of other joint and other extraarticular bone graft
W61 Fusion of other joint and other articular bone graft
W62 Other primary fusion of other joint
W63 Revisional fusion of other joint
W64 Conversion to fusion of other joint
W65 Primary open reduction of traumatic dislocation of joint
W66 Primary closed reduction of traumatic dislocation of joint
W67 Secondary reduction of traumatic dislocation of joint
W68 Primary reduction of injury to growth plate
W69 Open operations on synovial membrane of joint
W70 Open operations on semilunar cartilage
W71 Other open operations on intraarticular structure
W72 Prosthetic replacement of ligament
W73 Prosthetic reinforcement of ligament
W74 Other reconstruction of ligament
W75 Other open repair of ligament
W76 Other operations on ligament
W77 Stabilising operations on joint
W78 Release of contracture of joint
W79 Soft tissue operations on joint of toe
W81 Other open operations on joint
W82 Therapeutic endoscopic operations on semilunar cartilage
W83 Therapeutic endoscopic operations on other articular cartilage
W84 Therapeutic endoscopic operations on other joint structure
W85 Therapeutic endoscopic operations on cavity of knee joint
W86 Therapeutic endoscopic operations on cavity of other joint
W87 Diagnostic endoscopic examination of knee joint
W88 Diagnostic endoscopic examination of other joint
W90 Puncture of joint
W91 Other manipulation of joint
W92 Other operations on joint

X. MISCELLANEOUS OPERATIONS

Operations covering multiple systems (X01-X27)

X01 Replantation of upper limb
X02 Replantation of lower limb
X03 Replantation of other organ
X04 Transplantation between systems
X05 Implantation of prosthesis for limb
X07 Amputation of arm
X08 Amputation of hand
X09 Amputation of leg
X10 Amputation of foot
X11 Amputation of toe
X12 Operations on amputation stump
X14 Clearance of pelvis
X15 Operations for sexual transformation
X17 Separation of conjoined twins
X19 Correction of congenital deformity of shoulder or upper arm
X20 Correction of congenital deformity of forearm
X21 Correction of congenital deformity of hand
X22 Correction of congenital deformity of hip
X23 Correction of congenital deformity of leg
X24 Primary correction of congenital deformity of foot
X25 Other correction of congenital deformity of foot
X27 Correction of minor congenital deformity of foot

Miscellaneous operations (X29-X59)

X29 Continuous infusion of therapeutic substance
X30 Injection of therapeutic substance
X31 Injection of radiocontrast material
X32 Exchange blood transfusion
X33 Other blood transfusion
X34 Other intravenous transfusion
X35 Other intravenous injection
X36 Blood withdrawal
X37 Intramuscular injection
X38 Subcutaneous injection
X40 Compensation for renal failure
X41 Placement of ambulatory apparatus for compensation for renal failure
X42 Placement of other apparatus for compensation for renal failure
X45 Donation of organ
X46 Donation of other tissue
X48 Immobilisation using plaster cast
X49 Other immobilisation
X50 External resuscitation
X51 Change of body temperature
X53 Extirpation of unspecified organ
X55 Other operations on unspecified organ
X59 Anaesthetic without surgery

Y. SUBSIDIARY CLASSIFICATION OF METHODS OF OPERATION

Methods of operation not otherwise classifiable (Y01-Y44)

Y01 Replacement of organ noc
Y02 Placement of prosthesis in organ noc
Y03 Attention to prosthesis in organ noc
Y04 Replantation of organ noc
Y05 Excision of organ noc
Y06 Excision of lesion of organ noc
Y07 Obliteration of cavity of organ noc
Y08 Laser therapy to organ noc
Y09 Chemical destruction of organ noc
Y11 Other destruction of organ noc
Y12 Chemical destruction of lesion of organ noc
Y13 Other destruction of lesion of organ noc
Y16 Connection of organ noc
Y18 Release of organ noc
Y20 Other biopsy of organ noc
Y21 Cytology of organ noc
Y22 Drainage of organ noc
Y24 Microvascular repair of organ noc
Y25 Suture of organ noc
Y26 Other repair of organ noc
Y27 Graft to organ noc
Y29 Removal of foreign body from organ noc
Y30 Incision of organ noc
Y31 Exploration of organ noc
Y32 Reexploration of organ noc
Y33 Puncture of organ noc
Y35 Introduction of removable radioactive material into organ noc
Y36 Introduction of non removable material into organ noc
Y38 Injection of therapeutic inclusion substance into organ noc
Y39 Injection of other substance into organ noc
Y40 Dilation of organ noc
Y41 Examination of organ noc
Y42 Manipulation of organ noc
Y44 Other methods of operation on organ noc

Approach to organ (Y46-Y53)

Y46 Open approach to contents of cranium
Y47 Burrhole approach to contents of cranium
Y48 Approach to spine through back
Y49 Approach through thoracic cavity
Y50 Approach through abdominal cavity
Y51 Approach to organ through artificial opening into gastrointestinal tract
Y52 Approach to organ through other artificial opening
Y53 Percutaneous approach to organ under image control

Harvest of organ (Y54-Y69)

Y54 Harvest of nerve
Y55 Harvest of random pattern flap of skin from limb
Y56 Harvest of random pattern flap of skin from other site
Y57 Harvest of axial pattern flap of skin
Y58 Harvest of skin for graft
Y59 Harvest of flap of skin and fascia
Y60 Other harvest of fascia
Y61 Harvest of flap of skin and muscle of trunk
Y62 Harvest of flap of skin and muscle of other site
Y63 Harvest of flap of muscle of trunk
Y64 Harvest of flap of muscle of other site
Y65 Harvest of tendon
Y66 Harvest of bone
Y67 Harvest of other multiple tissue
Y69 Harvest of other tissue

Anaesthetic etc (Y70-Y90)

Y70 Early operations noc
Y71 Late operations noc
Y73 Facilitating operations noc
Y80 General anaesthetic
Y81 Spinal anaesthetic
Y82 Local anaesthetic
Y84 Other anaesthetic
Y90 Other nonoperations

Z. SUBSIDIARY CLASSIFICATION OF SITES OF OPERATION

Nervous system (Z01-Z12)

Z01 Tissue of brain
Z02 Ventricle of brain
Z03 Upper cranial nerve
Z04 Other cranial nerve
Z05 Meninges of brain
Z06 Spinal cord
Z07 Spinal nerve root
Z08 Brachial plexus
Z09 Peripheral nerve of arm
Z10 Lumbar plexus
Z11 Sacral plexus
Z12 Other nerve

Endocrine breast and special senses (Z13-Z21)

Z13   Endocrine gland of neck
Z14   Other endocrine gland
Z15   Breast
Z16   External structure of eye
Z17   Muscle of eye
Z18   Anterior chamber of eye
Z19   Other part of eye
Z20   Outer ear
Z21   Other part of ear

Respiratory tract and mouth (Z22-Z26)

Z22   Nose
Z23   Nasal sinus
Z24   Other respiratory tract
Z25   Mouth
Z26   Salivary apparatus

Digestive tract and abdominal organs (Z27-Z31)

Z27   Upper digestive tract
Z28   Large intestine
Z29   Other part of bowel
Z30   Biliary tract
Z31   Other abdominal organ

Heart arteries and veins (Z32-Z40)

Z32   Valve of heart
Z33   Other part of heart
Z34   Aorta
Z35   Cerebral artery
Z36   Branch of thoracic aorta
Z37   Lateral branch of abdominal aorta
Z38   Terminal branch of aorta
Z39   Vein
Z40   Other vascular tissue

Urinary tract and male genital organs (Z41-Z43)

Z41   Upper urinary tract
Z42   Lower urinary tract
Z43   Male genital organ

Female genital tract (Z44-Z46)

Z44   Vagina
Z45   Uterus
Z46   Other female genital tract

Skin (Z47-Z51)

Z47   Skin of face
Z48   Skin of other part of head or neck
Z49   Skin of trunk
Z50   Skin of other site
Z51   Nail

Soft tissue (Z52-Z62)

Z52   Chest wall
Z53   Abdominal wall
Z54   Muscle of shoulder or upper arm
Z55   Muscle of forearm
Z56   Muscle of hand
Z57   Muscle of hip or thigh
Z58   Muscle of lower leg
Z59   Muscle of foot
Z60   Other muscle
Z61   Lymph node
Z62   Other soft tissue

Bones and joints of skull and spine (Z63-Z67)

Z63   Bone of cranium
Z64   Bone of face
Z65   Jaw
Z66   Vertebra
Z67   Intervertebral joint

Other bones and joints (Z68-Z87)

Z68   Bone of shoulder girdle
Z69   Humerus
Z70   Radius
Z71   Ulna
Z72   Other bone of arm or wrist
Z73   Other bone of hand
Z74   Rib cage
Z75   Bone of pelvis
Z76   Femur
Z77   Tibia
Z78   Other bone of lower leg
Z79   Bone of tarsus
Z80   Other bone of foot
Z81   Joint of shoulder girdle or arm
Z82   Joint of wrist or hand
Z83   Joint of finger
Z84   Joint of pelvis or upper leg
Z85   Joint of lower leg or tarsus
Z86   Other joint of foot
Z87   Other part of musculoskeletal system

Other sites (Z89-Z94)

Z89   Arm region
Z90   Leg region
Z92   Other region of body
Z94   Laterality of operation

TABULAR LIST OF FOUR DIGIT SUBCATEGORIES

CHAPTER A

NERVOUS SYSTEM

(CODES A01-A84)

Excludes: ANAESTHETIC PROCEDURES (Chapter Y)

A01   Major excision of tissue of brain

A01.1   Hemispherectomy
A01.2   Total lobectomy of brain
A01.3   Partial lobectomy of brain
A01.8   Other specified
A01.9   Unspecified

A02   Excision of lesion of tissue of brain

A02.1   Excision of lesion of tissue of frontal lobe of brain
A02.2   Excision of lesion of tissue of temporal lobe of brain
A02.3   Excision of lesion of tissue of parietal lobe of brain
A02.4   Excision of lesion of tissue of occipital lobe of brain
A02.5   Excision of lesion of tissue of cerebellum
A02.8   Other specified
A02.9   Unspecified

A03   Stereotactic ablation of tissue of brain

A03.1   Stereotactic leucotomy
A03.2   Stereotactic ablation of tissue of thalamus
A03.3   Stereotactic ablation of tissue of globus pallidus
A03.4   Stereotactic ablation of tissue of brain stem
A03.8   Other specified
A03.9   Unspecified

A04   Open biopsy of lesion of tissue of brain
Includes: Tissue of brain

A04.1   Open biopsy of lesion of tissue of frontal lobe of brain
A04.2   Open biopsy of lesion of tissue of temporal lobe of brain
A04.3   Open biopsy of lesion of tissue of parietal lobe of brain
A04.4   Open biopsy of lesion of tissue of occipital lobe of brain
A04.5   Open biopsy of lesion of tissue of cerebellum
A04.6   Open biopsy of lesion of tissue of brain stem
A04.8   Other specified
A04.9   Unspecified

A05   Drainage of lesion of tissue of brain
Excludes: Drainage of subarachnoid space of brain (A22.1)
*   Drainage of extradural space (A40)*

A05.1   Drainage of abscess of tissue of brain
A05.2   Evacuation of haematoma from temporal lobe of brain
A05.3   Evacuation of haematoma from cerebellum
A05.4   Evacuation of intracerebral haematoma nec
A05.8   Other specified
A05.9   Unspecified

A07 **Other open operations on tissue of brain**

A07.1   Open division of tissue of brain
A07.2   Removal of foreign body from tissue of brain
A07.3   Exploration of tissue of brain
A07.8   Other specified
A07.9   Unspecified

A08 **Other biopsy of lesion of tissue of brain**
Includes: Tissue of brain

A08.1   Biopsy of lesion of tissue of frontal lobe of brain nec
A08.2   Biopsy of lesion of tissue of temporal lobe of brain nec
A08.3   Biopsy of lesion of tissue of parietal lobe of brain nec
A08.4   Biopsy of lesion of tissue of occipital lobe of brain nec
A08.5   Biopsy of lesion of tissue of cerebellum nec
A08.6   Biopsy of lesion of tissue of brain stem nec
A08.8   Other specified
A08.9   Unspecified

A09 **Neurostimulation of brain**

A09.1   Implantation of neurostimulator into brain
A09.2   Maintenance of neurostimulator in brain
A09.3   Removal of neurostimulator from brain
A09.8   Other specified
A09.9   Unspecified

A10 **Other operations on tissue of brain**

A10.1   Leucotomy nec
A10.2   Aspiration of abscess of tissue of brain
A10.3   Aspiration of haematoma of tissue of brain
A10.4   Aspiration of lesion of tissue of brain nec
A10.5   Puncture of tissue of brain nec
A10.8   Other specified
A10.9   Unspecified

A12 **Creation of connection from ventricle of brain**

A12.1   Ventriculocisternostomy
A12.2   Creation of ventriculovascular anastomosis
A12.3   Creation of ventriculopleural shunt
A12.4   Creation of ventriculoperitoneal shunt
A12.5   Creation of subcutaneous cerebrospinal fluid reservoir
A12.8   Other specified
A12.9   Unspecified

A13 **Attention to component of connection from ventricle of brain**

A13.1   Maintenance of proximal catheter of cerebroventricular shunt
A13.2   Maintenance of distal catheter of cerebroventricular shunt
A13.3   Insertion of antisyphon device into cerebroventricular shunt
A13.4   Renewal of valve of cerebroventricular shunt
A13.8   Other specified
A13.9   Unspecified

A14 Other operations on connection from ventricle of brain

A14.1 Renewal of cerebroventricular shunt
A14.2 Revision of cerebroventricular shunt nec
     Includes: Conversion of cerebroventricular shunt nec
A14.3 Removal of cerebroventricular shunt
A14.4 Irrigation of cerebroventricular shunt
A14.5 Attention to cerebroventricular shunt nec
A14.8 Other specified
A14.9 Unspecified

A16 Other open operations on ventricle of brain

A16.1 Open drainage of ventricle of brain nec
A16.8 Other specified
A16.9 Unspecified

A17 Therapeutic endoscopic operations on ventricle of brain
     Note: It is not necessary to code additionally any mention of diagnostic endoscopic examination of ventricle of brain (A18.9)

A17.1 Endoscopic extirpation of lesion of ventricle of brain
A17.8 Other specified
A17.9 Unspecified

A18 Diagnostic endoscopic examination of ventricle of brain

A18.1 Diagnostic endoscopic examination of ventricle of brain and biopsy of lesion of ventricle of brain
     Includes: Diagnostic endoscopic examination of ventricle of brain and biopsy of ventricle of brain
               Endoscopic biopsy of lesion of brain
               Endoscopic biopsy of brain
A18.8 Other specified
A18.9 Unspecified
     Includes: Ventriculoscopy of brain nec

A20 Other operations on ventricle of brain

A20.1 Drainage of ventricle of brain nec
A20.2 Ventriculography of brain
A20.3 Monitoring of pressure in ventricle of brain
A20.8 Other specified
A20.9 Unspecified

A22 Operations on subarachnoid space of brain

A22.1 Drainage of subarachnoid space of brain
A22.2 Puncture of cistern of brain
A22.3 Isotopic cisternography
A22.8 Other specified
A22.9 Unspecified

A24 Graft to cranial nerve

A24.1 Primary microsurgical graft to facial nerve (vii)
A24.2 Secondary microsurgical graft to facial nerve (vii)
A24.3 Microsurgical graft to facial nerve (vii) nec
A24.4 Primary microsurgical graft to cranial nerve nec
A24.5 Secondary microsurgical graft to cranial nerve nec
A24.6 Microsurgical graft to cranial nerve nec
A24.8 Other specified
A24.9 Unspecified

A25   **Intracranial transection of cranial nerve**

A25.1   Intracranial transection of optic nerve (ii)
A25.2   Intracranial transection of oculomotor nerve (iii)
        Includes: Intracranial transection of trochlear nerve (iv)
                 Intracranial transection of abducens nerve (vi)
A25.3   Intracranial transection of trigeminal nerve (v)
A25.4   Intracranial transection of facial nerve (vii)
A25.5   Intracranial transection of acoustic nerve (viii)
A25.6   Intracranial transection of glossopharyngeal nerve (ix)
A25.7   Intracranial transection of vagus nerve (x)
A25.8   Intracranial transection of specified cranial nerve nec
        Includes: Intracranial transection of accessory nerve (xi)
                 Intracranial transection of hypoglossal nerve (xii)
A25.9   Unspecified

A26   **Other intracranial destruction of cranial nerve**

A26.1   Intracranial destruction of optic nerve (ii)
A26.2   Intracranial destruction of oculomotor nerve (iii)
        Includes: Intracranial destruction of trochlear nerve (iv)
                 Intracranial destruction of abducens nerve (vi)
A26.3   Intracranial destruction of trigeminal nerve (v)
        Includes: Intracranial destruction of trigeminal ganglion
A26.4   Intracranial destruction of facial nerve (vii)
A26.5   Intracranial destruction of acoustic nerve (viii)
A26.6   Intracranial destruction of glossopharyngeal nerve (ix)
A26.7   Intracranial destruction of vagus nerve (x)
A26.8   Intracranial destruction of specified cranial nerve nec
        Includes: Intracranial destruction of accessory nerve (xi)
                 Intracranial destruction of hypoglossal nerve (xii)
A26.9   Unspecified

A27   **Extracranial extirpation of vagus nerve (x)**

A27.1   Extracranial truncal vagotomy
        Includes: Truncal vagotomy
A27.2   Proximal gastric vagotomy
        Includes: Highly selective vagotomy
                 Parietal cell vagotomy
A27.3   Selective extracranial vagotomy nec
        Includes: Selective vagotomy nec
A27.8   Other specified
A27.9   Unspecified
        Includes: Extracranial vagotomy nec
                 Vagotomy nec

A28   **Extracranial extirpation of other cranial nerve**

A28.1   Extracranial transection of trigeminal nerve (v) nec
        Includes: Transection of trigeminal nerve (v) nec
        Excludes: Neurectomy of vidian nerve (E12.4)
A28.2   Extracranial transection of accessory nerve (xi) nec
        Includes: Transection of accessory nerve (xi) nec
A28.8   Other specified
A28.9   Unspecified

A29   Excision of lesion of cranial nerve

A29.1   Excision of lesion of optic nerve (ii)
A29.2   Excision of lesion of oculomotor nerve (iii)
         Includes: Excision of lesion of trochlear nerve (iv)
                   Excision of lesion of abducens nerve (vi)
A29.3   Excision of lesion of trigeminal nerve (v)
A29.4   Excision of lesion of facial nerve (vii)
A29.5   Excision of lesion of acoustic nerve (viii)
A29.6   Excision of lesion of glossopharyngeal nerve (ix)
A29.7   Excision of lesion of vagus nerve (x)
A29.8   Excision of lesion of specified cranial nerve nec
         Includes: Excision of lesion of accessory nerve (xi)
                   Excision of lesion of hypoglossal nerve (xii)
A29.9   Unspecified

A30   Repair of cranial nerve

A30.1   Repair of optic nerve (ii)
A30.2   Repair of oculomotor nerve (iii)
         Includes: Repair of trochlear nerve (iv)
                   Repair of abducens nerve (vi)
A30.3   Repair of trigeminal nerve (v)
A30.4   Repair of facial nerve (vii)
A30.5   Repair of acoustic nerve (viii)
A30.6   Repair of glossopharyngeal nerve (ix)
A30.7   Repair of vagus nerve (x)
A30.8   Repair of specified cranial nerve nec
         Includes: Repair of accessory nerve (xi)
                   Repair of hypoglossal nerve (xii)
A30.9   Unspecified

A31   Intracranial stereotactic release of cranial nerve

A31.1   Intracranial stereotactic neurolysis of optic nerve (ii)
A31.2   Intracranial stereotactic neurolysis of oculomotor nerve (iii)
         Includes: Intracranial stereotactic neurolysis of trochlear nerve (iv)
                   Intracranial stereotactic neurolysis of abducens nerve (vi)
A31.3   Intracranial stereotactic neurolysis of trigeminal nerve (v)
A31.4   Intracranial stereotactic neurolysis of facial nerve (vii)
A31.5   Intracranial stereotactic neurolysis of acoustic nerve (viii)
A31.6   Intracranial stereotactic neurolysis of glossopharyngeal nerve (ix)
A31.7   Intracranial stereotactic neurolysis of vagus nerve (x)
A31.8   Intracranial stereotactic neurolysis of specified cranial nerve nec
         Includes: Intracranial stereotactic neurolysis of accessory nerve (xi)
                   Intracranial stereotactic neurolysis of hypoglossal nerve (xii)
A31.9   Unspecified

A32   Other decompression of cranial nerve

A32.1   Decompression of optic nerve (ii)
A32.2   Decompression of oculomotor nerve (iii)
         Includes: Decompression of trochlear nerve (iv)
                   Decompression of abducens nerve (vi)
A32.3   Decompression of trigeminal nerve (v)
A32.4   Decompression of facial nerve (vii)
A32.5   Decompression of acoustic nerve (viii)
A32.6   Decompression of glossopharyngeal nerve (ix)
A32.7   Decompression of vagus nerve (x)
A32.8   Decompression of specified cranial nerve nec
         Includes: Decompression of accessory nerve (xi)
                   Decomression of hypoglossal nerve (xii)
A32.9   Unspecified

A33   **Neurostimulation of cranial nerve**

A33.1   Introduction of neurostimulator into cranial nerve
A33.2   Maintenance of neurostimulator in cranial nerve
A33.3   Removal of neurostimulator from cranial nerve
A33.8   Other specified
A33.9   Unspecified

A34   **Exploration of cranial nerve**

A34.1   Exploration of optic nerve (ii)
A34.2   Exploration of oculomotor nerve (iii)
        Includes: Exploration of trochlear nerve (iv)
        Exploration of abducens nerve (vi)
A34.3   Exploration of trigeminal nerve (v)
A34.4   Exploration of facial nerve (vii)
A34.5   Exploration of acoustic nerve (viii)
A34.6   Exploration of glossopharyngeal nerve (ix)
A34.7   Exploration of vagus nerve (x)
A34.8   Exploration of specified cranial nerve nec
        Includes: Exploration of accessory nerve (xi)
        Exploration of hypoglossal nerve (xii)
A34.9   Unspecified

A36   **Other operations on cranial nerve**

A36.1   Hypoglossofacial anastomosis
A36.2   Anastomosis of cranial nerve nec
A36.3   Biopsy of lesion of cranial nerve
        Includes: Biopsy of cranial nerve
A36.8   Other specified
A36.9   Unspecified

A38   **Extirpation of lesion of meninges of brain**

A38.1   Extirpation of lesion of meninges of cortex of brain
A38.2   Extirpation of lesion of meninges of sphenoidal ridge of cranium
A38.3   Extirpation of lesion of meninges of subfrontal region of brain
A38.4   Extirpation of lesion of meninges of parasagittal region of brain
A38.5   Extirpation of lesion of falx cerebri
A38.6   Extirpation of lesion of tentorium cerebelli
A38.8   Other specified
A38.9   Unspecified

A39   **Repair of dura**

A39.1   Repair of meningoencephalocele
A39.2   Repair of dura of anterior fossa of cranium
A39.3   Repair of dura of middle fossa of cranium
A39.4   Repair of dura of posterior fossa of cranium
A39.5   Repair of dura of vault of cranium
A39.8   Other specified
A39.9   Unspecified

A40   **Drainage of extradural space**

A40.1   Evacuation of extradural haematoma
A40.8   Other specified
A40.9   Unspecified

A41   Drainage of subdural space

A41.1   Evacuation of subdural haematoma
A41.2   Drainage of abscess of subdural space
A41.8   Other specified
A41.9   Unspecified

A42   Other operations on meninges of brain

A42.1   Creation of anastomosis of dura
A42.2   Biopsy of lesion of meninges of brain
        Includes: Biopsy of meninges of brain
A42.8   Other specified
A42.9   Unspecified

A44   Partial extirpation of spinal cord

A44.1   Chordectomy of spinal cord
A44.2   Extirpation of lesion of spinal cord
A44.8   Other specified
A44.9   Unspecified

A45   Other open operations on spinal cord
        Includes: Spinal tract

A45.1   Stereotactic chordotomy of spinal cord
A45.2   Open chordotomy of spinal cord nec
A45.3   Myelotomy of spinal cord
A45.4   Open biopsy of lesion of spinal cord
        Includes: Open biopsy of spinal cord
A45.5   Removal of foreign body from spinal cord
A45.8   Other specified
A45.9   Unspecified

A47   Other destruction of spinal cord

A47.1   Needle destruction of substantia gelatinosa of cervical spinal cord
A47.2   Radiofrequency controlled thermal destruction of spinothalamic tract
A47.3   Percutaneous chordotomy of spinal cord
A47.8   Other specified
A47.9   Unspecified

A48   Other operations on spinal cord

A48.1   Biopsy of lesion of spinal cord nec
        Includes: Biopsy of spinal cord nec
A48.2   Aspiration of lesion of spinal cord
A48.3   Insertion of neurostimulator adjacent to spinal cord
A48.4   Attention to neurostimulator adjacent to spinal cord
A48.8   Other specified
A48.9   Unspecified

A49   Repair of spina bifida

A49.1   Freeing of spinal tether
A49.2   Closure of spinal myelomeningocele
A49.3   Closure of spinal meningocele
A49.8   Other specified
A49.9   Unspecified

A51   Other operations on meninges of spinal cord

A51.1   Extirpation of lesion of meninges of spinal cord
A51.2   Freeing of adhesions of meninges of spinal cord
A51.3   Biopsy of lesion of meninges of spinal cord
        Includes: Biopsy of meninges of spinal cord
A51.8   Other specified
A51.9   Unspecified

A52   Therapeutic epidural injection
        Excludes: Epidural anaesthetic procedures (Y81)

A52.1   Therapeutic lumbar epidural injection
A52.2   Therapeutic sacral epidural injection
A52.8   Other specified
A52.9   Unspecified

A53   Drainage of spinal canal

A53.1   Cerebrospinal syringostomy
A53.2   Creation of thecoperitoneal shunt
A53.3   Creation of syringoperitoneal shunt
A53.4   Creation of lumboperitoneal shunt
A53.5   Drainage of cerebrospinal fluid nec
A53.8   Other specified
A53.9   Unspecified

A54   Therapeutic spinal puncture

A54.1   Injection of destructive substance into cerebrospinal fluid
A54.2   Injection of therapeutic substance into cerebrospinal fluid
A54.8   Other specified
A54.9   Unspecified

A55   Diagnostic spinal puncture

A55.1   Radiculography
A55.2   Spinal myelography nec
A55.3   Spinal manometry
A55.8   Other specified
A55.9   Unspecified

A57   Operations on spinal nerve root
        Includes: Spinal nerve root ganglion

A57.1   Extirpation of lesion of spinal nerve root
A57.2   Rhizotomy of spinal nerve root
A57.3   Radiofrequency controlled thermal destruction of spinal nerve root
A57.4   Injection of destructive substance into spinal nerve root
A57.5   Destruction of spinal nerve root nec
A57.8   Other specified
A57.9   Unspecified

A59   Excision of peripheral nerve

A59.1   Total sacrifice of peripheral nerve
A59.2   Partial sacrifice of peripheral nerve
A59.8   Other specified
A59.9   Unspecified
        Includes: Neurectomy nec

A60 Destruction of peripheral nerve

A60.1 Enucleation of peripheral nerve
A60.2 Avulsion of peripheral nerve
A60.3 Transection of peripheral nerve
A60.4 Radiofrequency controlled thermal destruction of peripheral nerve
A60.5 Injection of destructive substance into peripheral nerve
A60.8 Other specified
A60.9 Unspecified

A61 Extirpation of lesion of peripheral nerve

A61.1 Excision of lesion of peripheral nerve
A61.2 Cryotherapy to lesion of peripheral nerve
A61.3 Radiotherapy to lesion of peripheral nerve
A61.4 Destruction of lesion of peripheral nerve nec
A61.8 Other specified
A61.9 Unspecified

A62 Microsurgical repair of peripheral nerve

A62.1 Primary microsurgical graft to peripheral nerve
A62.2 Secondary microsurgical graft to peripheral nerve
A62.3 Microsurgical graft to peripheral nerve nec
A62.4 Primary microsurgical repair of peripheral nerve nec
A62.5 Secondary microsurgical repair of peripheral nerve nec
A62.8 Other specified
A62.9 Unspecified

A63 Other graft to peripheral nerve

A63.1 Primary graft to peripheral nerve nec
A63.2 Secondary graft to peripheral nerve nec
A63.8 Other specified
A63.9 Unspecified

A64 Other repair of peripheral nerve

A64.1 Primary approximation of peripheral nerve
A64.2 Primary repair of peripheral nerve nec
A64.3 Secondary repair of peripheral nerve and mobilisation of peripheral nerve
A64.4 Secondary repair of peripheral nerve nec
A64.8 Other specified
A64.9 Unspecified

A65 Release of entrapment of peripheral nerve at wrist

A65.1 Carpal tunnel release
A65.2 Canal of guyon release
A65.8 Other specified
A65.9 Unspecified

A66 Release of entrapment of peripheral nerve at ankle

A66.1 Tarsal tunnel release
A66.8 Other specified
A66.9 Unspecified

A67   **Release of entrapment of peripheral nerve at other site**

A67.1   Cubital tunnel release
A67.2   Release of entrapment of lateral cutaneous nerve of thigh
A67.3   Release of entrapment of plantar digital nerve
A67.8   Other specified
A67.9   Unspecified

A68   **Other release of peripheral nerve**

A68.1   Primary neurolysis of peripheral nerve and transposition of peripheral nerve
A68.2   Secondary neurolysis of peripheral nerve and transposition of peripheral nerve
A68.3   Neurolysis of peripheral nerve and transposition of peripheral nerve nec
A68.4   Primary neurolysis of peripheral nerve nec
A68.5   Secondary neurolysis of peripheral nerve nec
A68.8   Other specified
A68.9   Unspecified
          Includes: Neurolysis of peripheral nerve nec

A69   **Revision of release of peripheral nerve**

A69.1   Revision of neurolysis of peripheral nerve and transposition of peripheral nerve
A69.8   Other specified
A69.9   Unspecified

A70   **Neurostimulation of peripheral nerve**

A70.1   Implantation of neurostimulator into peripheral nerve
A70.2   Maintenance of neurostimulator in peripheral nerve
A70.3   Removal of neurostimulator from peripheral nerve
A70.8   Other specified
A70.9   Unspecified

A73   **Other operations on peripheral nerve**

A73.1   Biopsy of lesion of peripheral nerve
          Includes: Biopsy of peripheral nerve
A73.2   Freeing of adhesions of peripheral nerve nec
A73.3   Decompression of peripheral nerve nec
A73.4   Exploration of peripheral nerve
A73.5   Injection of therapeutic substance around peripheral nerve
A73.8   Other specified
A73.9   Unspecified

A75   **Excision of sympathetic nerve**

A75.1   Excision of cervical sympathetic nerve
A75.2   Excision of thoracic sympathetic nerve
A75.3   Excision of lumbar sympathetic nerve
A75.4   Excision of perivascular sympathetic nerve
A75.5   Excision of splanchnic sympathetic nerve
A75.8   Other specified
A75.9   Unspecified
          Includes: Sympathectomy nec

A76   **Chemical destruction of sympathetic nerve**

A76.1   Chemical destruction of cervical sympathetic nerve
A76.2   Chemical destruction of thoracic sympathetic nerve
A76.3   Chemical destruction of lumbar sympathetic nerve
A76.4   Chemical destruction of perivascular sympathetic nerve
A76.5   Chemical destruction of splanchnic sympathetic nerve
A76.8   Other specified
A76.9   Unspecified
           Includes: Chemical sympathectomy nec

A77   **Cryotherapy to sympathetic nerve**

A77.1   Cryotherapy to cervical sympathetic nerve
A77.2   Cryotherapy to thoracic sympathetic nerve
A77.3   Cryotherapy to lumbar sympathetic nerve
A77.4   Cryotherapy to perivascular sympathetic nerve
A77.5   Cryotherapy to splanchnic sympathetic nerve
A77.8   Other specified
A77.9   Unspecified

A78   **Radiofrequency controlled thermal destruction of sympathetic nerve**

A78.1   Radiofrequency controlled thermal destruction of cervical sympathetic nerve
A78.2   Radiofrequency controlled thermal destruction of thoracic sympathetic nerve
A78.3   Radiofrequency controlled thermal destruction of lumbar sympathetic nerve
A78.4   Radiofrequency controlled thermal destruction of perivascular sympathetic nerve
A78.5   Radiofrequency controlled thermal destruction of splanchnic sympathetic nerve
A78.8   Other specified
A78.9   Unspecified

A79   **Other destruction of sympathetic nerve**

A79.1   Destruction of cervical sympathetic nerve nec
A79.2   Destruction of thoracic sympathetic nerve nec
A79.3   Destruction of lumbar sympathetic nerve nec
A79.4   Destruction of perivascular sympathetic nerve nec
A79.5   Destruction of splanchnic sympathetic nerve nec
A79.8   Other specified
A79.9   Unspecified

A81   **Other operations on sympathetic nerve**

A81.8   Other specified
A81.9   Unspecified

A83   **Electroconvulsive therapy**

A83.8   Other specified
A83.9   Unspecified

A84   **Neurophysiological operations**

A84.1   Electroencephalography
A84.2   Electromyography
A84.3   Nerve conduction studies
A84.4   Evoked potential recording
A84.5   Electroretinography
A84.8   Other specified
A84.9   Unspecified

CHAPTER B

ENDOCRINE SYSTEM AND BREAST

(CODES B01-B37)

B01 **Excision of pituitary gland**

B01.1 Transethmoidal hypophysectomy
B01.2 Transphenoidal hypophysectomy
B01.3 Transseptal hypophysectomy
B01.4 Transcranial hypophysectomy
B01.8 Other specified
B01.9 Unspecified
Includes: Hypophysectomy nec

B02 **Destruction of pituitary gland**

B02.1 Cryotherapy to pituitary gland
B02.2 Implantation of radioactive substance into pituitary gland
B02.3 Injection of destructive substance into pituitary gland nec
B02.8 Other specified
B02.9 Unspecified

B04 **Other operations on pituitary gland**
Includes: Pituitary stalk (B04.5)

B04.1 Excision of lesion of pituitary gland
B04.2 Biopsy of lesion of pituitary gland
Includes: Biopsy of pituitary gland
B04.3 Decompression of pituitary gland
B04.4 Exploration of pituitary gland
B04.5 Operations on pituitary stalk
B04.8 Other specified
B04.9 Unspecified

B06 **Operations on pineal gland**

B06.1 Excision of pineal gland
B06.8 Other specified
B06.9 Unspecified

B08 **Excision of thyroid gland**

B08.1 Total thyroidectomy
B08.2 Subtotal thyroidectomy
B08.3 Hemithyroidectomy
B08.4 Lobectomy of thyroid gland nec
B08.5 Isthmectomy of thyroid gland
B08.6 Partial thyroidectomy nec
B08.8 Other specified
B08.9 Unspecified
Includes: Thyroidectomy nec

B09 **Operations on aberrant thyroid tissue**

B09.1 Excision of substernal thyroid tissue
B09.2 Excision of sublingual thyroid tissue
B09.8 Other specified
B09.9 Unspecified

B10   Operations on thyroglossal tissue

B10.1   Excision of thyroglossal cyst
B10.2   Excision of thyroglossal tract
B10.3   Biopsy of lesion of thyroglossal tract
        Includes: Biopsy of thyroglossal tract
B10.4   Incision of thyroglossal cyst
B10.8   Other specified
B10.9   Unspecified

B12   Other operations on thyroid gland

B12.1   Excision of lesion of thyroid gland
B12.2   Biopsy of lesion of thyroid gland
        Includes: Biopsy of thyroid gland
B12.3   Incision of lesion of thyroid gland
B12.4   Exploration of thyroid gland
B12.8   Other specified
B12.9   Unspecified

B14   Excision of parathyroid gland

B14.1   Global parathyroidectomy and transposition of parathyroid tissue
B14.2   Global parathyroidectomy nec
B14.3   Partial parathyroidectomy and transposition of parathyroid tissue
B14.4   Partial parathyroidectomy nec
B14.5   Excision of lesion of parathyroid gland
B14.8   Other specified
B14.9   Unspecified
        Includes: Parathyroidectomy nec

B16   Other operations on parathyroid gland

B16.1   Modification of transposed parathyroid gland
B16.2   Biopsy of lesion of parathyroid gland
        Includes: Biopsy of parathyroid gland
B16.3   Exploration of parathyroid gland
B16.8   Other specified
B16.9   Unspecified

B18   Excision of thymus gland

B18.1   Transsternal thymectomy
B18.2   Transcervical thymectomy
B18.8   Other specified
B18.9   Unspecified
        Includes: Thymectomy nec

B20   Other operations on thymus gland

B20.1   Biopsy of lesion of thymus gland
        Includes: Biopsy of thymus gland
B20.2   Exploration of thymus gland
B20.8   Other specified
B20.9   Unspecified

B22   **Excision of adrenal gland**

B22.1   Bilateral adrenalectomy and transposition of adrenal tissue
B22.2   Bilateral adrenalectomy nec
B22.3   Unilateral adrenalectomy
         Includes: Adrenalectomy nec
B22.4   Partial adrenalectomy
B22.8   Other specified
B22.9   Unspecified

B23   **Operations on aberrant adrenal tissue**

B23.1   Excision of lesion of aberrant adrenal tissue
B23.2   Exploration of aberrant adrenal tissue
B23.8   Other specified
B23.9   Unspecified

B25   **Other operations on adrenal gland**

B25.1   Excision of lesion of adrenal gland
B25.2   Biopsy of lesion of adrenal gland
         Includes: Biopsy of adrenal gland
B25.3   Embolisation of adrenal gland
B25.4   Exploration of adrenal gland
B25.8   Other specified
B25.9   Unspecified

B27   **Total excision of breast**
        Note: *Use supplementary code for removal of lymph node (T85-T87)*
                 Radical mastectomy see Introduction page xi

B27.1   Total mastectomy and excision of both pectoral muscles and part of chest wall
B27.2   Total mastectomy and excision of both pectoral muscles nec
B27.3   Total mastectomy and excision of pectoralis minor muscle
B27.4   Total mastectomy nec
B27.5   Subcutaneous mastectomy
B27.8   Other specified
B27.9   Unspecified
         Includes: Mastectomy nec

B28   **Other excision of breast**
        Note: *Use supplementary code for removal of lymph node (T85-T87)*

B28.1   Quadrantectomy of breast
B28.2   Partial excision of breast nec
         Includes: Wedge excision of breast nec
B28.3   Excision of lesion of breast
         Includes: Lumpectomy of breast
B28.8   Other specified
B28.9   Unspecified

B29   **Reconstruction of breast**
        Note: *Use supplementary code for insertion of prosthesis for breast (B30.1)*

B29.1   Reconstruction of breast using myocutaneous flap of latissimus dorsi muscle
B29.2   Reconstruction of breast using local flap of skin nec
B29.3   Reconstruction of breast using flap of skin of abdomen
B29.4   Reconstruction of breast using distant flap of skin nec
B29.5   Revision of reconstruction of breast
B29.8   Other specified
B29.9   Unspecified

B30 **Prosthesis for breast**
Excludes: Augmentation mammoplasty (B31.2)

B30.1   Insertion of prosthesis for breast
B30.2   Revision of prosthesis for breast
B30.3   Removal of prosthesis for breast
B30.8   Other specified
B30.9   Unspecified

B31 **Other plastic operations on breast**

B31.1   Reduction mammoplasty
B31.2   Augmentation mammoplasty
B31.3   Mastopexy
B31.4   Revision of mammoplasty
B31.8   Other specified
B31.9   Unspecified

B32 **Biopsy of breast**

B32.1   Percutaneous biopsy of lesion of breast
         Includes: Percutaneous biopsy of breast
B32.2   Biopsy of lesion of breast nec
B32.8   Other specified
B32.9   Unspecified

B33 **Incision of breast**

B33.1   Drainage of lesion of breast
B33.2   Capsulotomy of breast
B33.3   Exploration of breast
B33.8   Other specified
B33.9   Unspecified

B34 **Operations on duct of breast**

B34.1   Subareolar excision of mammillary duct
B34.2   Excision of mammillary duct nec
B34.3   Excision of lesion of mammillary duct
B34.4   Microdochotomy
B34.5   Exploration of mammillary duct nec
B34.8   Other specified
B34.9   Unspecified

B35 **Operations on nipple**
Includes: Skin of nipple
Note: Codes from Chapter S may be used to enhance these codes

B35.1   Transposition of nipple
B35.2   Excision of nipple
B35.3   Extirpation of lesion of nipple
B35.4   Plastic operations on nipple
B35.5   Biopsy of lesion of nipple
         Includes: Biopsy of nipple
B35.6   Eversion of nipple
B35.8   Other specified
B35.9   Unspecified

B37 **Other operations on breast**

B37.1   Aspiration of lesion of breast
         Includes: Aspiration of breast
B37.2   Injection into breast
B37.3   Extraction of milk from breast
B37.8   Other specified
B37.9   Unspecified

CHAPTER C

EYE

(CODES C01-C86)

C01   **Excision of eye**
Note: *Use additional code as necessary for concurrent insertion of prosthetic replacement of eye (C03)*

C01.1   Exenteration of orbit
C01.2   Enucleation of eyeball
C01.3   Evisceration of contents of eyeball
C01.8   Other specified
C01.9   Unspecified

C02   **Extirpation of lesion of orbit**

C02.1   Excision of lesion of orbit
C02.2   Destruction of lesion of orbit
C02.8   Other specified
C02.9   Unspecified

C03   **Insertion of prosthesis of eye**
Note: *Use as secondary code when associated with concurrent excision of eye (C01)*

C03.1   Insertion of prosthetic replacement for orbit
C03.2   Insertion of prosthetic replacement for eyeball
C03.8   Other specified
C03.9   Unspecified

C04   **Attention to prosthesis of eye**

C04.1   Revision of prosthetic replacement for orbit
C04.2   Revision of prosthetic replacement for eyeball
C04.3   Removal of prosthetic replacement for orbit
C04.4   Removal of prosthetic replacement for eyeball
C04.8   Other specified
C04.9   Unspecified

C05   **Plastic repair of orbit**

C05.1   Reconstruction of cavity of orbit
C05.2   Plastic repair of cavity of orbit
C05.3   Enlargement of cavity of orbit
C05.8   Other specified
C05.9   Unspecified

C06   **Incision of orbit**

C06.1   Biopsy of lesion of orbit
          Includes: Biopsy of orbit
C06.2   Drainage of orbit
C06.3   Decompression of orbit
C06.4   Removal of foreign body from orbit
C06.5   Exploration of orbit
C06.8   Other specified
C06.9   Unspecified
          Includes: Orbitotomy nec

C08   Other operations on orbit

C08.1   Transposition of ligament of orbit
C08.2   Open reduction of fracture of orbit
C08.3   Removal of fixation from fracture of orbit
C08.4   Retroocular injection into orbit
C08.8   Other specified
C08.9   Unspecified

C10   Operations on eyebrow
Includes: Skin of eyebrow
Note: Codes from Chapter S may be used to enhance these codes

C10.1   Excision of lesion of eyebrow
C10.2   Hair bearing flap to eyebrow
C10.3   Hair bearing graft to eyebrow
C10.4   Suture of eyebrow
C10.5   Incision of lesion of eyebrow
C10.8   Other specified
C10.9   Unspecified

C11   Operations on canthus
Note: Codes from Chapter S may be used to enhance these codes

C11.1   Excision of lesion of canthus
C11.2   Destruction of lesion of canthus
C11.3   Correction of epicanthus
C11.4   Correction of telecanthus
C11.5   Graft of skin to canthus
C11.6   Canthotomy
C11.8   Other specified
C11.9   Unspecified

C12   Extirpation of lesion of eyelid
Includes: Skin of eyelid
Note: Codes from Chapter S may be used to enhance these codes

C12.1   Excision of lesion of eyelid
C12.2   Cauterisation of lesion of eyelid
C12.3   Cryotherapy to lesion of eyelid
C12.4   Curettage of lesion of eyelid
C12.5   Destruction of lesion of eyelid nec
C12.8   Other specified
C12.9   Unspecified

C13   Excision of redundant skin of eyelid

C13.1   Blepharoplasty of both eyelids
C13.2   Blepharoplasty of upper eyelid
C13.3   Blepharoplasty of lower eyelid
C13.4   Blepharoplasty nec
C13.8   Other specified
C13.9   Unspecified

C14   Reconstruction of eyelid

C14.1   Flap of skin to eyelid
C14.2   Graft of skin to eyelid
C14.8   Other specified
C14.9   Unspecified

C15 **Correction of deformity of eyelid**

C15.1 Correction of ectropion
C15.2 Correction of entropion
C15.3 Correction of trichiasis
C15.8 Other specified
C15.9 Unspecified

C16 **Other plastic repair of eyelid**

C16.1 Central tarsorrhaphy
C16.2 Lateral tarsorrhaphy
C16.3 Medial tarsorrhaphy
C16.4 Tarsorrhaphy nec
C16.5 Revision of tarsorrhaphy
C16.8 Other specified
C16.9 Unspecified

C17 **Other repair of eyelid**
    Note at C12 applies
    Includes: Skin of eyelid

C17.1 Suture of eyelid
    Excludes: Protective suture of eyelid (C20)
C17.8 Other specified
C17.9 Unspecified

C18 **Correction of ptosis of eyelid**

C18.1 Correction of ptosis of eyelid using levator muscle technique
C18.2 Correction of ptosis of eyelid using frontalis muscle technique
C18.3 Correction of ptosis of eyelid using sling of fascia
C18.4 Correction of ptosis of eyelid using superior rectus muscle technique
C18.5 Tarsomullerectomy
C18.6 Correction of ptosis of eyelid using aponeurosis technique
C18.8 Other specified
C18.9 Unspecified

C19 **Incision of eyelid**
    Note at C12 applies
    Includes: Skin of eyelid

C19.1 Drainage of lesion of eyelid
C19.8 Other specified
C19.9 Unspecified

C20 **Protective suture of eyelid**

C20.1 Complete protective suture of eyelid
C20.2 Central protective suture of eyelid
C20.3 Lateral protective suture of eyelid
C20.4 Medial protective suture of eyelid
C20.5 Removal of protective suture from eyelid
C20.8 Other specified
C20.9 Unspecified

C22 **Other operations on eyelid**
Note at C12 applies
Includes: Skin of eyelid

C22.1 Avulsion of nerve of eyelid
C22.2 Biopsy of lesion of eyelid
Includes: Biopsy of eyelid
C22.3 Removal of foreign body from eyelid
C22.4 Injection into eyelid
C22.5 Exploration of eyelid
C22.6 Epilation of eyelash
C22.8 Other specified
C22.9 Unspecified

C24 **Operations on lacrimal gland**

C24.1 Excision of lacrimal gland
C24.2 Radiotherapy to lacrimal gland
C24.3 Destruction of lacrimal gland nec
C24.4 Biopsy of lesion of lacrimal gland
Includes: Biopsy of lacrimal gland
C24.5 Incision of lacrimal gland
C24.8 Other specified
C24.9 Unspecified

C25 **Connection between lacrimal apparatus and nose**

C25.1 Canaliculodacryocystorhinostomy
C25.2 Conjunctivodacryocystorhinostomy
C25.3 Dacryocystorhinostomy and insertion of tube hfq
C25.4 Dacryocystorhinostomy nec
C25.5 Revision of anastomosis between lacrimal apparatus and nose
C25.8 Other specified
C25.9 Unspecified

C26 **Other operations on lacrimal sac**

C26.1 Excision of lacrimal sac
C26.2 Destruction of lesion of lacrimal sac
C26.3 Biopsy of lesion of lacrimal sac
Includes: Biopsy of lacrimal sac
C26.4 Incision of lacrimal sac
C26.8 Other specified
C26.9 Unspecified

C27 **Operations on nasolacrimal duct**

C27.1 Drainage of nasolacrimal duct
Includes: Insertion of tube into nasolacrimal duct
C27.2 Dilation of nasolacrimal duct
C27.3 Irrigation of nasolacrimal duct
Includes: Syringing of nasolacrimal duct
C27.4 Removal of tube from nasolacrimal duct
C27.5 Probing of nasolacrimal duct nec
C27.8 Other specified
C27.9 Unspecified

C29 Other operations on lacrimal apparatus

C29.1 Repair of canaliculus
C29.2 Enlargement of lacrimal punctum
C29.3 Occlusion of lacrimal punctum
C29.8 Other specified
C29.9 Unspecified

C31 Combined operations on muscles of eye

C31.1 Recession of medial rectus muscle and resection of lateral rectus muscle of eye
C31.2 Bilateral recession of medial recti muscles of eyes
C31.3 Bilateral resection of medial recti muscles of eyes
C31.4 Bilateral recession of lateral recti muscles of eyes
C31.5 Bilateral resection of lateral recti muscles of eyes
C31.8 Other specified
C31.9 Unspecified

C32 Recession of muscle of eye

C32.1 Recession of medial rectus muscle of eye nec
C32.2 Recession of lateral rectus muscle of eye nec
C32.3 Recession of superior rectus muscle of eye
C32.4 Recession of inferior rectus muscle of eye
C32.5 Recession of superior oblique muscle of eye
C32.6 Recession of inferior oblique muscle of eye
C32.7 Recession of combinations of muscles of eye
C32.8 Other specified
C32.9 Unspecified

C33 Resection of muscle of eye
Includes: Advancement of muscle of eye
Plication of muscle of eye
Tucking of muscle of eye

C33.1 Resection of medial rectus muscle of eye nec
C33.2 Resection of lateral rectus muscle of eye nec
C33.3 Resection of superior rectus muscle of eye
C33.4 Resection of inferior rectus muscle of eye
C33.5 Resection of superior oblique muscle of eye
C33.6 Resection of inferior oblique muscle of eye
C33.7 Resection of combinations of muscles of eye
C33.8 Other specified
C33.9 Unspecified

C34 Partial division of tendon of muscle of eye

C34.1 Tenotomy of medial rectus muscle of eye
C34.2 Tenotomy of lateral rectus muscle of eye
C34.3 Tenotomy of superior rectus muscle of eye
C34.4 Tenotomy of inferior rectus muscle of eye
C34.5 Tenotomy of superior oblique muscle of eye
C34.6 Tenotomy of inferior oblique muscle of eye
C34.7 Tenotomy of combinations of muscles of eye
C34.8 Other specified
C34.9 Unspecified
Includes: Tenotomy of muscle of eye nec

C35 Other adjustment to muscle of eye

C35.1 Transposition of muscle of eye nec
C35.2 Lengthening of muscle of eye by muscle slide
C35.3 Insertion of adjustable suture into muscle of eye
C35.8 Other specified
C35.9 Unspecified

C37 Other operations on muscle of eye

C37.1 Excision of lesion of muscle of eye
C37.2 Freeing of adhesions of muscle of eye
C37.3 Biopsy of lesion of muscle of eye
      Includes: Biopsy of muscle of eye
C37.4 Repair of muscle of eye nec
C37.8 Other specified
C37.9 Unspecified

C39 Extirpation of lesion of conjunctiva

C39.1 Excision of lesion of conjunctiva
C39.2 Cauterisation of lesion of conjunctiva
C39.3 Cryotherapy to lesion of conjunctiva
C39.4 Curettage of lesion of conjunctiva
C39.5 Radiotherapy to lesion of conjunctiva
C39.8 Other specified
C39.9 Unspecified

C40 Repair of conjunctiva

C40.1 Mucosal graft to conjunctiva
C40.2 Amniotic graft to conjunctiva
C40.3 Sliding graft to conjunctiva
C40.4 Prosthetic replacement of conjunctiva
C40.5 Suture of conjunctiva
C40.8 Other specified
C40.9 Unspecified

C41 Incision of conjunctiva

C41.1 Peritomy
C41.8 Other specified
C41.9 Unspecified

C43 Other operations on conjunctiva

C43.1 Division of adhesions of conjunctiva
C43.2 Biopsy of lesion of conjunctiva
      Includes: Biopsy of conjunctiva
C43.3 Removal of foreign body from conjunctiva
C43.4 Subconjunctival injection
C43.5 Exploration of conjunctiva
C43.6 Creation of hood of conjunctiva
C43.8 Other specified
C43.9 Unspecified

C45   Extirpation of lesion of cornea

C45.1   Superficial keratectomy
C45.2   Excision of lesion of cornea nec
C45.3   Cauterisation of lesion of cornea
C45.4   Cryotherapy to lesion of cornea
C45.5   Radiotherapy to lesion of cornea
C45.6   Destruction of lesion of cornea nec
C45.7   Debridement of lesion of cornea
C45.8   Other specified
C45.9   Unspecified

C46   Plastic operations on cornea

C46.1   Refractive keratoplasty
C46.2   Lamellar graft to cornea
C46.3   Penetrating graft to cornea
C46.4   Insertion of prosthesis into cornea
C46.8   Other specified
C46.9   Unspecified

C47   Closure of cornea

C47.1   Suture of cornea
C47.2   Adjustment to suture of cornea
C47.3   Removal of suture from cornea
C47.8   Other specified
C47.9   Unspecified

C48   Removal of foreign body from cornea

C48.1   Surgical removal of foreign body from cornea
C48.2   Magnetic extraction of foreign body from cornea
C48.8   Other specified
C48.9   Unspecified

C49   Incision of cornea

C49.1   Section of cornea
C49.2   Trephine of cornea
C49.3   Radial keratotomy
C49.8   Other specified
C49.9   Unspecified

C51   Other operations on cornea

C51.1   Biopsy of lesion of cornea
        Includes: Biopsy of cornea
C51.2   Chelation of cornea
C51.3   Exploration of cornea
C51.4   Tattooing of cornea
C51.8   Other specified
C51.9   Unspecified

C53   Extirpation of lesion of sclera

C53.1   Punch resection of sclera
C53.2   Excision of lesion of sclera nec
C53.3   Cauterisation of lesion of sclera
C53.4   Destruction of lesion of sclera nec
C53.8   Other specified
C53.9   Unspecified

C54   Buckling operations for attachment of retina

C54.1   Overlay scleroplasty
C54.2   Imbrication of sclera
C54.3   Buckling of sclera and implant hfq
C54.4   Buckling of sclera and local or encircling explant hfq
C54.5   Buckling of sclera nec
C54.6   Removal of implant or explant from sclera
C54.8   Other specified
C54.9   Unspecified

C55   Incision of sclera

C55.1   Drainage of lesion of sclera
C55.2   Corneoscleral trephine
C55.3   Drainage of subretinal fluid through sclera
C55.8   Other specified
C55.9   Unspecified
         Includes: Sclerotomy nec

C57   Other operations on sclera

C57.1   Biopsy of lesion of sclera
         Includes: Biopsy of sclera
C57.2   Repair of sclera
C57.3   Graft to sclera
C57.4   Suture of sclera
C57.8   Other specified
C57.9   Unspecified

C59   Excision of iris

C59.1   Iridocyclectomy
C59.2   Surgical iridectomy
         Includes: Iridectomy nec
C59.8   Other specified
C59.9   Unspecified

C60   Filtering operations on iris

C60.1   Trabeculectomy
C60.2   Inclusion of iris
C60.3   Fixation of iris
C60.4   Iridoplasty nec
         Includes: Pupilloplasty
C60.5   Insertion of tube into anterior chamber of eye to assist drainage of aqueous humour
C60.8   Other specified
C60.9   Unspecified

C61   Other operations on trabecular meshwork of eye

C61.1   Laser trabeculoplasty
C61.2   Trabeculotomy
C61.3   Goniotomy
C61.4   Goniopuncture
C61.8   Other specified
C61.9   Unspecified

C62 **Incision of iris**

C62.1 Iridosclerotomy
C62.2 Surgical iridotomy
Includes: Iridotomy nec
C62.3 Laser iridotomy
C62.4 Correction iridodialysis nec
C62.8 Other specified
C62.9 Unspecified

C64 **Other operations on iris**

C64.1 Excision of prolapsed iris
C64.2 Excision of lesion of iris
C64.3 Destruction of lesion of iris
C64.4 Biopsy of lesion of iris
Includes: Biopsy of iris
C64.5 Removal of foreign body from iris
C64.6 Stretching of iris
C64.8 Other specified
C64.9 Unspecified

C66 **Extirpation of ciliary body**

C66.1 Excision of ciliary body
Includes: Excision of lesion of ciliary body
C66.2 Cauterisation of ciliary body
C66.3 Cryotherapy to ciliary body
C66.4 Laser photocoagulation of ciliary body
C66.5 Destruction of ciliary body nec
C66.8 Other specified
C66.9 Unspecified

C67 **Other operations on ciliary body**

C67.1 Separation of ciliary body
Includes: Cyclodialysis
C67.8 Other specified
C67.9 Unspecified

C69 **Other operations on anterior chamber of eye**

C69.1 Reformation of anterior chamber of eye
C69.2 Paracentesis of anterior chamber of eye
C69.3 Injection into anterior chamber of eye
C69.4 Irrigation of anterior chamber of eye
Includes: Washout of anterior chamber of eye
C69.8 Other specified
C69.9 Unspecified

C71 **Extracapsular extraction of lens**
Note: *Use as additional code when associated with concurrent insertion of prosthetic replacement for lens (C75.1)*

C71.1 Simple linear extraction of lens
Includes: Needling of lens for cataract
C71.2 Phakoemulsification of lens
C71.3 Aspiration of lens
C71.8 Other specified
C71.9 Unspecified

C72 **Intracapsular extraction of lens**
Note: *Use as additional code when associated with concurrent insertion of prosthetic replacement for lens (C75.1)*

C72.1 Forceps extraction of lens
C72.2 Suction extraction of lens
C72.3 Cryoextraction of lens
C72.8 Other specified
C72.9 Unspecified

C73 **Incision of capsule of lens**
Note: *Use as additional code when associated with concurrent insertion of prosthetic replacement for lens (C75.1)*

C73.1 Membranectomy of lens
C73.2 Capsulotomy of anterior lens capsule
C73.3 Capsulotomy of posterior lens capsule
C73.4 Capsulotomy of lens nec
C73.8 Other specified
C73.9 Unspecified

C74 **Other extraction of lens**
Note: *Use as additional code when associated with concurrent insertion of prosthetic replacement for lens (C75.1)*

C74.1 Curettage of lens
C74.2 Discission of cataract
C74.3 Mechanical lensectomy
C74.8 Other specified
C74.9 Unspecified

C75 **Prosthesis of lens**
Note: *Use supplementary code to identify method of concurrent extraction of lens (C71-C74)*

C75.1 Insertion of prosthetic replacement for lens
C75.2 Revision of prosthetic replacement for lens
C75.3 Removal of prosthetic replacement for lens
C75.8 Other specified
C75.9 Unspecified

C77 **Other operations on lens**

C77.1 Capsulectomy
C77.2 Couching of lens
C77.3 Biopsy of lesion of lens
Includes: Biopsy of lens
C77.4 Surgical removal of foreign body from lens
C77.5 Magnetic extraction of foreign body from lens
C77.8 Other specified
C77.9 Unspecified

C79 **Operations on vitreous body**

C79.1 Extirpation of vitreous body using anterior approach
C79.2 Extirpation of vitreous body nec
C79.3 Injection of vitreous substitute into vitreous body
C79.4 Injection into vitreous body nec
C79.8 Other specified
C79.9 Unspecified

C81 Photocoagulation of retina for detachment

C81.1 Xenon photocoagulation of retina for detachment
C81.2 Laser photocoagulation of retina for detachment
C81.8 Other specified
C81.9 Unspecified

C82 Destruction of lesion of retina
Includes: Destruction of retina

C82.1 Cauterisation of lesion of retina
Includes: Photocoagulation of lesion of retina nec
Electrocoagulation of lesion of retina nec
C82.2 Cryotherapy to lesion of retina
C82.3 Radiotherapy to lesion of retina
C82.8 Other specified
C82.9 Unspecified

C84 Other operations on retina
Includes: Choroid

C84.1 Epiretinal dissection
C84.2 Excision of lesion of retina
C84.3 Biopsy of lesion of retina
Includes: Biopsy of retina
C84.8 Other specified
C84.9 Unspecified

C86 Other operations on eye

C86.1 Biopsy of lesion of eye nec
Includes: Biopsy of eye nec
C86.2 Repair of globe
Includes: Repair of penetrating injury to eye
C86.3 Suture of eye nec
C86.4 Removal of foreign body from eye nec
C86.5 Fluorescein angiography of eye
C86.6 Examination of eye under anaesthetic
C86.8 Other specified
C86.9 Unspecified

CHAPTER D

EAR

(CODES D01-D28)

D01   **Excision of external ear**

D01.1   Total excision of external ear
D01.2   Partial excision of external ear
D01.3   Excision of preauricular abnormality
D01.8   Other specified
D01.9   Unspecified

D02   **Extirpation of lesion of external ear**
Includes: Skin of external ear
Note: *Codes from Chapter S may be used to enhance these codes*

D02.1   Excision of lesion of external ear
D02.2   Destruction of lesion of external ear
D02.8   Other specified
D02.9   Unspecified

D03   **Plastic operations on external ear**
Note at D02 applies
Includes: Skin of external ear
Excludes: Replantation of ear (X03.1)

D03.1   Reconstruction of external ear using graft
D03.2   Reconstruction of external ear nec
D03.3   Pinnaplasty
       Includes: Correction of prominent ear
D03.4   Meatoplasty of external ear
D03.8   Other specified
D03.9   Unspecified

D04   **Drainage of external ear**
Note at D02 applies
Includes: Skin of external ear

D04.1   Drainage of haematoma of external ear
D04.2   Drainage of abscess of external ear
D04.8   Other specified
D04.9   Unspecified

D06   **Other operations on external ear**
Note at D02 applies
Includes: Skin of external ear

D06.1   Biopsy of lesion of external ear
       Includes: Biopsy of external ear
D06.2   Repair of lobe of external ear
D06.3   Repair of external ear nec
D06.8   Other specified
D06.9   Unspecified

D07   **Clearance of external auditory canal**

D07.1   Irrigation of external auditory canal for removal of wax
   Includes: Syringing of ear for removal of wax
      Washout of ear for removal of wax
D07.2   Removal of wax from external auditory canal nec
D07.3   Removal of foreign body from external auditory canal
D07.8   Other specified
D07.9   Unspecified

D08   **Other operations on external auditory canal**

D08.1   Extirpation of lesion of external auditory canal
D08.2   Reconstruction of external auditory canal
D08.3   Drainage of external auditory canal
D08.4   Incision of external auditory canal
D08.5   Irrigation of external auditory canal nec
D08.8   Other specified
D08.9   Unspecified

D10   **Exenteration of mastoid air cells**

D10.1   Radical mastoidectomy nec
D10.2   Modified radical mastoidectomy
D10.3   Cortical mastoidectomy
D10.4   Simple mastoidectomy
   Includes: Mastoidectomy nec
D10.5   Excision of lesion of mastoid
D10.6   Revision of mastoidectomy
D10.8   Other specified
D10.9   Unspecified

D12   **Other operations on mastoid**
   Includes: Attic

D12.1   Obliteration of mastoid
D12.2   Atticotomy
D12.3   Biopsy of mastoid
D12.4   Exploration of mastoid
D12.5   Removal of pack from mastoid
D12.8   Other specified
D12.9   Unspecified

D14   **Repair of eardrum**

D14.1   Tympanoplasty using graft
   Includes: Myringoplasty using graft
D14.2   Tympanoplasty nec
   Includes: Myringoplasty nec
D14.3   Revision of tympanoplasty
   Includes: Revision of myringoplasty
D14.8   Other specified
D14.9   Unspecified

D15　　**Drainage of middle ear**

D15.1　Insertion of ventilation tube through tympanic membrane
　　　　Includes: Insertion of grommet through tympanic membrane
D15.2　Suction clearance of middle ear
D15.3　Incision of ear drum nec
　　　　Includes: Myringotomy nec
　　　　　　　　Tympanotomy nec
　　　　　　　　Exploration of middle ear
D15.8　Other specified
D15.9　Unspecified

D16　　**Reconstruction of ossicular chain**

D16.1　Prosthetic replacement of ossicular chain
D16.2　Graft replacement of ossicular chain
D16.8　Other specified
D16.9　Unspecified

D17　　**Other operations on ossicle of ear**

D17.1　Stapedectomy
D17.2　Revision of stapedectomy
D17.3　Division of adhesions of ossicle of ear
D17.8　Other specified
D17.9　Unspecified

D19　　**Extirpation of lesion of middle ear**

D19.1　Excision of lesion of middle ear
D19.2　Destruction of lesion of middle ear
D19.8　Other specified
D19.9　Unspecified

D20　　**Other operations on middle ear**

D20.1　Biopsy of lesion of middle ear
　　　　Includes: Biopsy of middle ear
D20.2　Maintenance of ventilation tube through tympanic membrane
　　　　Includes: Maintenance of grommet through tympanic membrane
D20.3　Removal of ventilation tube from tympanic membrane
　　　　Includes: Removal of grommet from tympanic membrane
D20.8　Other specified
D20.9　Unspecified

D22　　**Operations on eustachian canal**

D22.1　Graft to eustachian canal
D22.2　Intubation of eustachian canal
D22.3　Insufflation of eustachian canal
D22.8　Other specified
D22.9　Unspecified

D24   **Operations on cochlea**

D24.1   Implantation of intracochlear prosthesis
D24.2   Implantation of extracochlear prosthesis
D24.3   Attention to cochlear prosthesis
D24.4   Neurectomy of cochlea
D24.5   Transtympanic electrocochleography
D24.8   Other specified
D24.9   Unspecified

D26   **Operations on vestibular apparatus**

D26.1   Operations on endolymphatic sac
D26.2   Membranous labyrinthectomy
D26.3   Osseous labyrinthectomy
D26.4   Neurectomy of vestibular apparatus
D26.8   Other specified
D26.9   Unspecified

D28   **Other operations on ear**

D28.1   Biopsy of lesion of ear nec
          Includes: Biopsy of ear nec
D28.2   Examination of ear under anaesthetic
D28.8   Other specified
D28.9   Unspecified

CHAPTER E

RESPIRATORY TRACT

(CODES E01-E63)

Excludes: CHEST WALL   (Chapter T)
                PLEURA   (Chapter T)
                PLEURAL CAVITY   (Chapter T)

E01   **Excision of nose**

E01.1   Total excision of nose
E01.8   Other specified
E01.9   Unspecified

E02   **Plastic operations on nose**
        Excludes: Replantation of nose (X03.2)
        Note: *Codes from Chapter S may be used to enhance these codes*

E02.1   Total reconstruction of nose
E02.2   Reconstruction of nose nec
E02.3   Septorhinoplasty using implant
E02.4   Septorhinoplasty using graft
E02.5   Reduction rhinoplasty
E02.6   Rhinoplasty nec
E02.8   Other specified
E02.9   Unspecified

E03   **Operations on septum of nose**

E03.1   Submucous excision of septum of nose
E03.2   Excision of lesion of septum of nose
E03.3   Biopsy of lesion of septum of nose
        Includes: Biopsy of septum of nose
E03.4   Closure of perforation of septum of nose
E03.5   Incision of septum of nose
E03.6   Septoplasty of nose nec
E03.8   Other specified
E03.9   Unspecified

E04   **Operations on turbinate of nose**

E04.1   Submucous diathermy to turbinate of nose
E04.2   Excision of turbinate of nose nec
        Includes: Reduction of turbinate of nose nec
E04.3   Excision of lesion of turbinate of nose nec
E04.4   Division of adhesions of turbinate of nose
E04.5   Biopsy of lesion of turbinate of nose
        Includes: Biopsy of turbinate of nose
E04.6   Cauterisation of turbinate of nose
E04.8   Other specified
E04.9   Unspecified

E05   **Surgical arrest of bleeding from internal nose**
Includes: Surgical arrest of spontaneous bleeding from internal nose

E05.1   Cauterisation of internal nose
E05.2   Ligation of artery of internal nose
E05.3   Embolisation of artery of internal nose
E05.8   Other specified
E05.9   Unspecified

E06   **Packing of cavity of nose**

E06.1   Packing of posterior cavity of nose
E06.2   Packing of anterior cavity of nose
E06.3   Removal of packing from cavity of nose
E06.8   Other specified
E06.9   Unspecified

E08   **Other operations on internal nose**

E08.1   Polypectomy of internal nose
E08.2   Extirpation of lesion of internal nose nec
E08.3   Correction of congenital atresia of choana
E08.4   Division of adhesions of internal nose
E08.5   Removal of foreign body from cavity of nose
E08.8   Other specified
E08.9   Unspecified

E09   **Operations on external nose**
Includes: Skin of external nose
Note: *Codes from Chapter S may be used to enhance these codes*

E09.1   Excision of lesion of external nose
E09.2   Destruction of lesion of external nose
E09.3   Suture of external nose
E09.4   Shave of skin of nose
E09.5   Biopsy of lesion of external nose
Includes: Biopsy of external nose
E09.8   Other specified
E09.9   Unspecified

E10   **Other operations on nose**

E10.1   Biopsy of lesion of nose nec
Includes: Biopsy of nose nec
E10.8   Other specified
E10.9   Unspecified

E12   **Operations on maxillary antrum using sublabial approach**

E12.1   Ligation of maxillary artery using sublabial approach
E12.2   Drainage of maxillary antrum using sublabial approach
E12.3   Irrigation of maxillary antrum using sublabial approach
Includes: Washout of maxillary antrum using sublabial approach
E12.4   Transantral neurectomy of vidian nerve using sublabial approach
E12.8   Other specified
E12.9   Unspecified

E13   **Other operations on maxillary antrum**

E13.1   Drainage of maxillary antrum nec
E13.2   Excision of lesion of maxillary antrum
E13.3   Intranasal antrostomy
E13.4   Biopsy of lesion of maxillary antrum
        Includes: Biopsy of maxillary antrum
E13.5   Closure of fistula between maxillary antrum and mouth
E13.6   Puncture of maxillary antrum
        Includes: Irrigation of maxillary antrum nec
E13.8   Other specified
E13.9   Unspecified

E14   **Operations on frontal sinus**
        Includes: Ethmoid sinus

E14.1   External frontoethmoidectomy
E14.2   Intranasal ethmoidectomy
E14.3   External ethmoidectomy
E14.4   Transantral ethmoidectomy
E14.5   Bone flap to frontal sinus
E14.6   Trephine of frontal sinus
E14.8   Other specified
E14.9   Unspecified

E15   **Operations on sphenoid sinus**

E15.1   Drainage of sphenoid sinus
E15.2   Puncture of sphenoid sinus
E15.8   Other specified
E15.9   Unspecified

E17   **Operations on unspecified nasal sinus**

E17.1   Excision of nasal sinus nec
E17.2   Excision of lesion of nasal sinus nec
E17.3   Biopsy of lesion of nasal sinus nec
        Includes: Biopsy of nasal sinus nec
E17.4   Lateral rhinotomy into nasal sinus nec
E17.8   Other specified
E17.9   Unspecified

E19   **Excision of pharynx**
        Includes: Nasopharynx

E19.1   Total pharyngectomy
E19.2   Partial pharyngectomy
        Includes: Pharyngectomy nec
E19.8   Other specified
E19.9   Unspecified

E20   **Operations on adenoid**

E20.1   Total adenoidectomy
        Includes: Excision of adenoid
                 Adenoidectomy
        Note: Use as secondary code when associated with excision of tonsil (F34)
E20.2   Biopsy of adenoid
        Includes: Biopsy of lesion of adenoid
E20.8   Other specified
E20.9   Unspecified

E21   **Repair of pharynx**
Includes: Nasopharynx

E21.1   Pharyngoplasty using posterior pharyngeal implant
E21.2   Pharyngoplasty using posterior pharyngeal flap
E21.3   Pharyngoplasty using lateral pharyngeal flap
E21.4   Plastic repair of pharynx nec
E21.8   Other specified
E21.9   Unspecified

E23   **Other open operations on pharynx**
Includes: Nasopharynx

E23.1   Open excision of lesion of pharynx
E23.2   Operations on pharyngeal pouch
E23.8   Other specified
E23.9   Unspecified

E24   **Therapeutic endoscopic operations on pharynx**
Includes: Nasopharynx
Note: ***It is not necessary to code additionally any mention of diagnostic endoscopic examination of nasopharynx (E25.3) or pharynx nec (E25.9)***

E24.1   Endoscopic extirpation of lesion of nasopharynx
E24.2   Endoscopic extirpation of lesion of pharynx nec
E24.8   Other specified
E24.9   Unspecified

E25   **Diagnostic endoscopic examination of pharynx**

E25.1   Diagnostic endoscopic examination of nasopharynx and biopsy of lesion of nasopharynx
Includes: Diagnostic endoscopic examination of nasopharynx and biopsy of nasopharynx
Endoscopic biopsy of lesion of nasopharynx
Endoscopic biopsy of nasopharynx
Biopsy of lesion of nasopharynx nec
Biopsy of nasopharynx nec
E25.2   Diagnostic endoscopic examination of pharynx and biopsy of lesion of pharynx nec
Includes: Diagnostic endoscopic examination of pharynx and biopsy of pharynx nec
Endoscopic biopsy of lesion of pharynx nec
Endoscopic biopsy of pharynx nec
Biopsy of lesion of pharynx nec
Biopsy of pharynx nec
E25.3   Diagnostic endoscopic examination of nasopharynx nec
Includes: Nasopharyngoscopy nec
E25.8   Other specified
E25.9   Unspecified
Includes: Pharyngoscopy nec

E27   **Other operations on pharynx**
Includes: Nasopharynx

E27.1   Open biopsy of lesion of pharynx
Includes: Open biopsy of pharynx
E27.2   Drainage of retropharyngeal abscess
E27.3   Incision of pharynx nec
E27.4   Removal of foreign body from pharynx
E27.5   Dilation of pharynx
E27.6   Examination of pharynx under anaesthetic
E27.8   Other specified
E27.9   Unspecified

E29   **Excision of larynx**

E29.1   Total laryngectomy
E29.2   Partial horizontal laryngectomy
E29.3   Partial vertical laryngectomy
E29.4   Partial laryngectomy nec
E29.5   Laryngofissure and chordectomy of vocal chord
E29.6   Laryngectomy nec
E29.8   Other specified
E29.9   Unspecified

E30   **Open extirpation of lesion of larynx**

E30.1   Excision of lesion of larynx using thyrotomy as approach
E30.2   Excision of lesion of larynx using lateral pharyngotomy as approach
E30.3   Open destruction of lesion of larynx
E30.8   Other specified
E30.9   Unspecified

E31   **Reconstruction of larynx**

E31.1   Laryngotracheal reconstruction using cartilage graft
E31.2   Laryngotracheoplasty nec
E31.3   Division of stenosis of larynx and insertion of prosthesis into larynx
E31.4   Implantation of artificial voice box into larynx
E31.5   Attention to artificial voice box in larynx
E31.8   Other specified
E31.9   Unspecified

E33   **Other open operations on larynx**

E33.1   External arytenoidectomy
E33.2   Chordopexy of vocal chord
E33.3   Operations on cartilage of larynx nec
       Includes: Chondroplasty of larynx
E33.4   Open biopsy of lesion of larynx
       Includes: Open biopsy of larynx
E33.8   Other specified
E33.9   Unspecified

E34   **Microtherapeutic endoscopic operations on larynx**
       Note: *It is not necessary to code additionally any mention of diagnostic endoscopic examination of larynx (E36.9)*

E34.1   Microtherapeutic endoscopic extirpation of lesion of larynx using laser
E34.2   Microtherapeutic endoscopic resection of lesion of larynx nec
E34.3   Microtherapeutic endoscopic destruction of lesion of larynx nec
E34.8   Other specified
E34.9   Unspecified

E35   **Other therapeutic endoscopic operations on larynx**
       Note: *It is not necessary to code additionally any mention of diagnostic endoscopic examination of larynx (E36.9)*

E35.1   Endoscopic arytenoidectomy
E35.2   Endoscopic resection of lesion of larynx
E35.3   Endoscopic destruction of lesion of larynx
E35.4   Endoscopic removal of prosthesis from larynx
E35.5   Endoscopic removal of foreign body from larynx
E35.8   Other specified
E35.9   Unspecified

E36   **Diagnostic endoscopic examination of larynx**

E36.1   Diagnostic endoscopic examination of larynx and biopsy of lesion of larynx
       Includes: Diagnostic endoscopic examination of larynx and biopsy of larynx
       Endoscopic biopsy of lesion of larynx
       Endoscopic biopsy of larynx
       Biopsy of lesion of larynx nec
       Biopsy of larynx nec
E36.8   Other specified
E36.9   Unspecified
       Includes: Laryngoscopy nec

E38   **Other operations on larynx**

E38.1   Injection into larynx
E38.8   Other specified
E38.9   Unspecified

E39   **Partial excision of trachea**
       Note: Use additional code for excision of carina as necessary (E44.1)

E39.1   Open excision of lesion of trachea
       Includes: Excision of lesion of trachea nec
E39.8   Other specified
E39.9   Unspecified

E40   **Plastic operations on trachea**
       Note: Use additional code for reconstruction of carina as necessary (E44.1)

E40.1   Reconstruction of trachea and anastomosis hfq
E40.2   Reconstruction of trachea using graft
E40.3   Reconstruction of trachea nec
E40.8   Other specified
E40.9   Unspecified

E41   **Open placement of prosthesis in trachea**
       Excludes: Placement of tracheostomy tube (E42)

E41.1   Open insertion of tubal prosthesis in trachea
E41.2   Open renewal of tubal prosthesis in trachea
E41.3   Open removal of tubal prosthesis from trachea
E41.8   Other specified
E41.9   Unspecified

E42   **Exteriorisation of trachea**

E42.1   Permanent tracheostomy
E42.2   Cricothyroidostomy
E42.3   Temporary tracheostomy
       Includes: Tracheostomy nec
       Tracheotomy
       Placement of tracheostomy tube
E42.4   Revision of tracheostomy
E42.5   Closure of tracheostomy
E42.6   Replacement of tracheostomy tube
E42.7   Removal of tracheostomy tube
E42.8   Other specified
E42.9   Unspecified

E43   Other open operations on trachea

E43.1   Open destruction of lesion of trachea
E43.2   Tracheorrhaphy
E43.3   Tracheopexy
E43.4   Open biopsy of lesion of trachea
         Includes: Open biopsy of trachea
E43.8   Other specified
E43.9   Unspecified

E44   Open operations on carina

E44.1   Excision of carina
         Excludes: When associated with reconstruction of carina (E44.2)
         Note: Use as secondary code in association with excision of trachea (E39) bronchus (E46) or lung
         (E54) as necessary
E44.2   Reconstruction of carina
         Includes: Excision of carina and reconstruction hfq
         Note: Use as secondary code in association with plastic operations on trachea (E40)
E44.3   Open biopsy of lesion of carina
         Includes: Open biopsy of carina
E44.8   Other specified
E44.9   Unspecified

E45   Code deleted

E46   Partial extirpation of bronchus
         Note: Use additional code for excision of carina as necessary (E44.1)

E46.1   Sleeve resection of bronchus and anastomosis hfq
E46.2   Excision of cyst of bronchus
E46.3   Excision of lesion of bronchus nec
E46.4   Open destruction of lesion of bronchus
E46.8   Other specified
E46.9   Unspecified

E47   Other open operations on bronchus

E47.1   Open biopsy of lesion of bronchus nec
         Includes: Open biopsy of bronchus nec
E47.2   Closure of fistula of bronchus
E47.3   Repair of bronchus nec
E47.8   Other specified
E47.9   Unspecified

E48   Therapeutic fibreoptic endoscopic operations on lower respiratory tract
         Includes: Trachea
                   Carina
                   Bronchus
                   Lung
         Note: It is not necessary to code additionally any mention of diagnostic fibreoptic endoscopic
         examination of lower respiratory tract (E49.9)
         Use subsidiary site code as necessary

E48.1   Fibreoptic endoscopic snare resection of lesion of lower respiratory tract
E48.2   Fibreoptic endoscopic laser destruction of lesion of lower respiratory tract
E48.3   Fibreoptic endoscopic destruction of lesion of lower respiratory tract nec
E48.4   Fibreoptic endoscopic aspiration of lower respiratory tract
E48.5   Fibreoptic endoscopic removal of foreign body from lower respiratory tract
E48.6   Fibreoptic endoscopic irrigation of lower respiratory tract
         Includes: Fibreoptic endoscopic lavage of lower respiratory tract
E48.8   Other specified
E48.9   Unspecified

E49 **Diagnostic fibreoptic endoscopic examination of lower respiratory tract**
Includes: Trachea
Carina
Bronchus
Lung
Note: ***Use subsidiary site code as necessary***

E49.1 Diagnostic fibreoptic endoscopic examination of lower respiratory tract and biopsy of lesion of lower respiratory tract
Includes: Diagnostic fibreoptic endoscopic examination of lower respiratory tract and biopsy of lower respiratory tract
Fibreoptic endoscopic biopsy of lesion of lower respiratory tract
Fibreoptic endoscopic biopsy of lower respiratory tract
E49.8 Other specified
E49.9 Unspecified
Includes: Fibreoptic bronchoscopy nec

E50 **Therapeutic endoscopic operations on lower respiratory tract using rigid bronchoscope**
Includes: Therapeutic endoscopic operations on lower respiratory tract nec
Trachea
Carina
Bronchus
Lung
Note: ***It is not necessary to code additionally any mention of diagnostic endoscopic examination of lower respiratory tract using rigid bronchoscope (E51.9)***
Use subsidiary site code as necessary

E50.1 Endoscopic snare resection of lesion of lower respiratory tract using rigid bronchoscope
E50.2 Endoscopic laser destruction of lesion of lower respiratory tract using rigid bronchoscope
E50.3 Endoscopic destruction of lesion of lower respiratory tract using rigid bronchoscope nec
E50.4 Endoscopic aspiration of lower respiratory tract using rigid bronchoscope
E50.5 Endoscopic removal of foreign body from lower respiratory tract using rigid bronchoscope
E50.6 Endoscopic irrigation of lower respiratory tract using rigid bronchoscope
Includes: Endoscopic lavage of lower respiratory tract using rigid bronchoscope
E50.8 Other specified
E50.9 Unspecified

E51 **Diagnostic endoscopic examination of lower respiratory tract using rigid bronchoscope**
Includes: Diagnostic therapeutic endoscopic examination of lower respiratory tract nec
Trachea
Carina
Bronchus
Lung
Note: ***Use subsidiary site code as necessary***

E51.1 Diagnostic endoscopic examination of lower respiratory tract and biopsy of lesion of lower respiratory tract using rigid bronchoscope
Includes: Diagnostic endoscopic examination of lower respiratory tract and biopsy of lower respiratory tract using rigid bronchoscope
Endoscopic biopsy of lesion of lower respiratory tract using rigid bronchoscope
Endoscopic biopsy of lower respiratory tract using rigid bronchoscope
Biopsy of lesion of lower respiratory tract nec
Biopsy of lower respiratory tract nec
Excludes: Biopsy of lesion of lung nec (E59)
Biopsy of lung nec (E59)
E51.8 Other specified
E51.9 Unspecified
Includes: Tracheoscopy nec
Bronchoscopy nec
Tracheobronchoscopy nec

E52   **Other operations on bronchus**
        Includes: Trachea

E52.1   Irrigation of bronchus nec
        Includes: Lavage of bronchus nec
E52.2   Aspiration of bronchus nec
        Includes: Clearance of airway
E52.8   Other specified
E52.9   Unspecified

E53   **Transplantation of lung**
        Excludes: Transplantation of heart and lung (K01)

E53.8   Other specified
E53.9   Unspecified

E54   **Excision of lung**
        Note: Use additional code for excision of carina as necessary (E44.1)

E54.1   Total pneumonectomy
        Includes: Pneumonectomy nec
E54.2   Bilobectomy of lung
E54.3   Lobectomy of lung
E54.4   Excision of segment of lung
E54.5   Partial lobectomy of lung nec
E54.8   Other specified
E54.9   Unspecified

E55   **Open extirpation of lesion of lung**

E55.1   Open decortication of lesion of lung
E55.2   Open excision of lesion of lung
        Includes: Excision of lesion of lung nec
E55.3   Open cauterisation of lesion of lung
E55.4   Open destruction of lesion of lung nec
E55.8   Other specified
E55.9   Unspecified

E57   **Other open operations on lung**

E57.1   Repair of lung
E57.2   Ligation of bulla of lung
E57.3   Deflation of bulla of lung
E57.4   Incision of lung nec
E57.8   Other specified
E57.9   Unspecified

E59   **Other operations on lung**

E59.1   Needle biopsy of lesion of lung
        Includes: Needle biopsy of lung
E59.2   Aspiration biopsy of lesion of lung
        Includes: Aspiration biopsy of lung
E59.3   Biopsy of lesion of lung nec
        Includes: Biopsy of lung nec
E59.4   Drainage of lung
E59.8   Other specified
E59.9   Unspecified

E61   **Open operations on mediastinum**

E61.1   Open excision of lesion of mediastinum
E61.2   Open biopsy of lesion of mediastinum
        Includes: Open biopsy of mediastinum
E61.3   Open drainage of mediastinum
E61.4   Mediastinotomy nec
E61.5   Exploration of mediastinum nec
E61.8   Other specified
E61.9   Unspecified

E62   **Therapeutic endoscopic operations on mediastinum**
        Note: ***It is not necessary to code additionally any mention of diagnostic endoscopic examination of mediastinum (E63.9)***

E62.1   Endoscopic extirpation of lesion of mediastinum
E62.8   Other specified
E62.9   Unspecified

E63   **Diagnostic endoscopic examination of mediastinum**

E63.1   Diagnostic endoscopic examination of mediastinum and biopsy of lesion of mediastinum
        Includes: Diagnostic endoscopic examination of mediastinum and biopsy of mediastinum
               Endoscopic biopsy of lesion of mediastinum
               Endoscopic biopsy of mediastinum
               Biopsy of lesion of mediastinum nec
               Biopsy of mediastinum nec
E63.8   Other specified
E63.9   Unspecified
        Includes: Cervical mediastinoscopy nec
               Mediastinoscopy nec

CHAPTER F

MOUTH

(CODES F01-F58)

F01   **Partial excision of lip**
Includes: Skin of lip
Note: **Codes from Chapter S may be used to enhance these codes**

F01.1   Excision of vermilion border of lip and advancement of mucosa of lip
F01.8   Other specified
F01.9   Unspecified

F02   **Extirpation of lesion of lip**
Note at F01 applies
Includes: Skin of lip
           Mucosa of lip

F02.1   Excision of lesion of lip
F02.2   Destruction of lesion of lip
F02.8   Other specified
F02.9   Unspecified

F03   **Correction of deformity of lip**
Note at F01 applies
Includes: Skin of lip

F03.1   Primary closure of cleft lip
F03.2   Revision of primary closure of cleft lip
F03.3   Adjustment to vermilion border of lip nec
F03.8   Other specified
F03.9   Unspecified

F04   **Other reconstruction of lip**
Note at F01 applies
Includes: Skin of lip

F04.1   Reconstruction of lip using tongue flap
F04.2   Reconstruction of lip using skin flap
F04.8   Other specified
F04.9   Unspecified

F05   **Other repair of lip**
Note at F01 applies
Includes: Skin of lip

F05.1   Excision of excess mucosa from lip
F05.2   Advancement of mucosa of lip nec
F05.3   Suture of lip
F05.8   Other specified
F05.9   Unspecified

F06   **Other operations on lip**
Note at F01 applies
Includes: Skin of lip
Mucosa of lip

F06.1   Division of adhesions of lip
F06.2   Biopsy of lesion of lip
Includes: Biopsy of lip
F06.3   Shave of lip
F06.8   Other specified
F06.9   Unspecified

F08   **Implantation of tooth**

F08.1   Allotransplantation of tooth
F08.2   Autotransplantation of tooth
F08.3   Replantation of tooth
F08.4   Repositioning of tooth
F08.8   Other specified
F08.9   Unspecified

F09   **Surgical removal of tooth**

F09.1   Surgical removal of impacted wisdom tooth
F09.2   Surgical removal of impacted tooth nec
F09.3   Surgical removal of wisdom tooth nec
F09.4   Surgical removal of tooth nec
F09.5   Surgical removal of retained root of tooth
F09.8   Other specified
F09.9   Unspecified

F10   **Simple extraction of tooth**

F10.1   Full dental clearance
Includes: Dental clearance nec
F10.2   Upper dental clearance
F10.3   Lower dental clearance
F10.4   Extraction of multiple teeth nec
F10.8   Other specified
F10.9   Unspecified
Includes: Extraction of single tooth

F11   **Preprosthetic oral surgery**
Excludes: Reduction of fracture of alveolus (V08 V15)

F11.1   Oral alveoplasty
F11.2   Augmentation of alveolar ridge using autobone graft
F11.3   Augmentation of alveolar ridge nec
F11.4   Vestibuloplasty of mouth
F11.5   Endosseous implantation into jaw
F11.6   Subperiosteal implantation into jaw
F11.8   Other specified
F11.9   Unspecified

F12   **Surgery on apex of tooth**

F12.1   Apicectomy of tooth
F12.2   Root canal therapy to tooth
F12.8   Other specified
F12.9   Unspecified

F13 Restoration of tooth

F13.1 Full restoration of crown of tooth
F13.2 Partial restoration of crown of tooth
F13.3 Restoration of crown of tooth nec
F13.4 Restoration of part of tooth using inlay nec
F13.5 Restoration of part of tooth using filling nec
F13.8 Other specified
F13.9 Unspecified

F14 Orthodontic operations

F14.1 Insertion of fixed orthodontic appliance
F14.2 Insertion of movable orthodontic appliance
F14.3 Insertion of orthodontic appliance nec
F14.4 Removal of orthodontic appliance
F14.5 Surgical exposure of tooth
F14.8 Other specified
F14.9 Unspecified

F16 Other operations on tooth

F16.1 Drainage of abscess of alveolus of tooth
F16.2 Surgical arrest of postoperative bleeding from tooth socket
F16.3 Packing of tooth socket
F16.4 Scaling of tooth
F16.8 Other specified
F16.9 Unspecified

F18 Excision of dental lesion of jaw

F18.1 Enucleation of dental cyst of jaw
F18.2 Marsupialisation of dental lesion of jaw
F18.8 Other specified
F18.9 Unspecified

F20 Operations on gingiva

F20.1 Excision of gingiva
Includes: Gingivectomy nec
F20.2 Excision of lesion of gingiva
F20.3 Biopsy of lesion of gingiva
Includes: Biopsy of gingiva
F20.4 Gingivoplasty
F20.5 Suture of gingiva
F20.8 Other specified
F20.9 Unspecified

F22 Excision of tongue

F22.1 Total glossectomy
F22.2 Partial glossectomy
F22.8 Other specified
F22.9 Unspecified
Includes: Glossectomy nec

F23   **Extirpation of lesion of tongue**

F23.1   Excision of lesion of tongue
F23.2   Destruction of lesion of tongue
F23.8   Other specified
F23.9   Unspecified

F24   **Incision of tongue**

F24.1   Biopsy of lesion of tongue
        Includes: Biopsy of tongue
F24.2   Removal of foreign body from tongue
F24.3   Glossotomy
F24.8   Other specified
F24.9   Unspecified

F26   **Other operations on tongue**

F26.1   Commissurectomy of tongue
F26.2   Excision of frenulum of tongue
F26.3   Incision of frenulum of tongue
        Includes: Frenotomy of tongue
F26.4   Freeing of adhesions of tongue
F26.5   Suture of tongue
F26.8   Other specified
F26.9   Unspecified

F28   **Extirpation of lesion of palate**

F28.1   Excision of lesion of palate
F28.2   Destruction of lesion of palate
F28.8   Other specified
F28.9   Unspecified

F29   **Correction of deformity of palate**

F29.1   Primary repair of cleft palate
F29.2   Revision of repair of cleft palate
F29.8   Other specified
F29.9   Unspecified

F30   **Other repair of palate**

F30.1   Plastic repair of palate using flap of palate
F30.2   Plastic repair of palate using flap of skin
F30.3   Plastic repair of palate using flap of tongue
F30.4   Plastic repair of palate using graft of skin
F30.5   Plastic repair of palate using flap of mucosa
F30.6   Plastic repair of palate using graft of mucosa
F30.7   Suture of palate
F30.8   Other specified
F30.9   Unspecified

F32   **Other operations on palate**
        Includes: Uvula (F32.4)

F32.1   Biopsy of lesion of palate
        Includes: Biopsy of palate
F32.2   Removal of foreign body from palate
F32.3   Incision of palate
F32.4   Operations on uvula
F32.8   Other specified
F32.9   Unspecified

F34   **Excision of tonsil**
        Note: *Use supplementary code for concurrent excision of adenoid (E20.1)*

F34.1   Bilateral dissection tonsillectomy
F34.2   Bilateral guillotine tonsillectomy
F34.3   Bilateral laser tonsillectomy
F34.4   Bilateral excision of tonsil nec
        Includes: Bilateral tonsillectomy nec
F34.5   Excision of remnant of tonsil
F34.6   Excision of lingual tonsil
F34.8   Other specified
F34.9   Unspecified
        Includes: Tonsillectomy nec

F36   **Other operations on tonsil**
        Includes: Peritonsillar region

F36.1   Destruction of tonsil
        Includes: Destruction of lesion of tonsil
F36.2   Biopsy of lesion of tonsil
        Includes: Biopsy of tonsil
F36.3   Drainage of abscess of peritonsillar region
F36.4   Removal of foreign body from tonsil
F36.5   Surgical arrest of postoperative bleeding from tonsillar bed
F36.8   Other specified
F36.9   Unspecified

F38   **Extirpation of lesion of other part of mouth**
        Includes: Unspecified part of mouth

F38.1   Excision of lesion of floor of mouth
F38.2   Excision of lesion of mouth nec
F38.3   Destruction of lesion of floor of mouth
F38.4   Destruction of lesion of mouth nec
F38.8   Other specified
F38.9   Unspecified

F39   **Reconstruction of other part of mouth**
        Includes: Unspecified part of mouth

F39.1   Reconstruction of mouth using flap nec
F39.2   Reconstruction of mouth using graft nec
F39.8   Other specified
F39.9   Unspecified

F40   **Other repair of other part of mouth**
        Includes: Unspecified part of mouth

F40.1   Revision of repair of mouth nec
F40.2   Graft of skin to mouth nec
F40.3   Graft of mucosa to mouth nec
F40.4   Suture of mouth nec
F40.8   Other specified
F40.9   Unspecified

F42   Other operations on mouth

F42.1   Biopsy of lesion of mouth nec
        Includes: Biopsy of mouth nec
F42.2   Incision of mouth nec
F42.3   Removal of excess mucosa from mouth nec
F42.8   Other specified
F42.9   Unspecified

F44   Excision of salivary gland

F44.1   Total excision of parotid gland
F44.2   Partial excision of parotid gland
F44.3   Excision of parotid gland nec
F44.4   Excision of submandibular gland
F44.5   Excision of sublingual gland
F44.8   Other specified
F44.9   Unspecified

F45   Extirpation of lesion of salivary gland

F45.1   Excision of lesion of parotid gland
F45.2   Excision of lesion of submandibular gland
F45.3   Excision of lesion of sublingual gland
F45.4   Excision of lesion of salivary gland nec
F45.5   Destruction of lesion of salivary gland
F45.8   Other specified
F45.9   Unspecified

F46   Incision of salivary gland

F46.1   Incision of parotid gland
F46.2   Incision of submandibular gland
F46.3   Incision of sublingual gland
F46.8   Other specified
F46.9   Unspecified

F48   Other operations on salivary gland

F48.1   Biopsy of lesion of salivary gland
        Includes: Biopsy of salivary gland
F48.2   Closure of fistula of salivary gland
F48.3   Repair of salivary gland nec
F48.4   Sialography
F48.8   Other specified
F48.9   Unspecified

F50   Transposition of salivary duct

F50.1   Transposition of parotid duct
F50.2   Transposition of submandibular duct
F50.8   Other specified
F50.9   Unspecified

F51   Open extraction of calculus from salivary duct

F51.1   Open extraction of calculus from parotid duct
F51.2   Open extraction of calculus from submandibular duct
F51.8   Other specified
F51.9   Unspecified

F52   Ligation of salivary duct

F52.1   Ligation of parotid duct
F52.2   Ligation of submandibular duct
F52.8   Other specified
F52.9   Unspecified

F53   Other open operations on salivary duct

F53.1   Open operations on parotid duct nec
F53.2   Open operations on submandibular duct nec
F53.8   Other specified
F53.9   Unspecified

F55   Dilation of salivary duct

F55.1   Dilation of parotid duct
F55.2   Dilation of submandibular duct
F55.8   Other specified
F55.9   Unspecified

F55   Manipulative removal of calculus from salivary duct

F56.1   Manipulative removal of calculus from parotid duct
F56.2   Manipulative removal of calculus from submandibular duct
F56.8   Other specified
F56.9   Unspecified

F58   Other operations on salivary duct

F58.1   Operations on parotid duct nec
F58.2   Operations on submandibular duct nec
F58.8   Other specified
F58.9   Unspecified

CHAPTER G

UPPER DIGESTIVE TRACT

(CODES G01-G82)

G01   Excision of oesophagus and stomach

G01.1   Oesophagogastrectomy and anastomosis of oesophagus to stomach
G01.2   Oesophagogastrectomy and anastomosis of oesophagus to transpose jejunum
G01.3   Oesophagogastrectomy and anastomosis of oesophagus to jejunum nec
G01.8   Other specified
G01.9   Unspecified

G02   Total excision of oesophagus

G02.1   Total oesophagectomy and anastomosis of pharynx to stomach
G02.2   Total oesophagectomy and interposition of microvascularly attached jejunum
G02.3   Total oesophagectomy and interposition of jejunum nec
G02.4   Total oesophagectomy and interposition of microvascularly attached colon
G02.5   Total oesophagectomy and interposition of colon nec
G02.8   Other specified
G02.9   Unspecified

G03   Partial excision of oesophagus

G03.1   Partial oesophagectomy and end to end anastomosis of oesophagus
          Includes: Partial oesophagectomy and reanastomosis of oesophagus to stomach
G03.2   Partial oesophagectomy and interposition of microvascularly attached jejunum
G03.3   Partial oesophagectomy and anastomosis of oesophagus to transposed jejunum
G03.4   Partial oesophagectomy and anastomosis of oesophagus to jejunum nec
G03.5   Partial oesophagectomy and interposition of microvascularly attached colon
G03.6   Partial oesophagectomy and interposition of colon nec
G03.8   Other specified
G03.9   Unspecified
          Includes: Oesophagectomy nec

G04   Open extirpation of lesion of oesophagus

G04.1   Excision of lesion of oesophagus
G04.2   Open laser destruction of lesion of oesophagus
G04.3   Open destruction of lesion of oesophagus nec
G04.8   Other specified
G04.9   Unspecified

G05   Bypass of oesophagus
          Includes: Anastomosis or interposition of oesophagus without mention of bypass
          Excludes: When associated with excision of oesophagus   (G01-G03)

G05.1   Bypass of oesophagus by anastomosis of oesophagus to oesophagus
G05.2   Bypass of oesophagus by anastomosis of oesophagus to stomach
G05.3   Bypass of oesophagus by interposition of microvascularly attached jejunum
G05.4   Bypass of oesophagus by interposition of jejunum nec
G05.5   Bypass of oesophagus by interposition of microvascularly attached colon
G05.6   Bypass of oesophagus by interposition of colon nec
G05.8   Other specified
G05.9   Unspecified

G06   **Attention to connection of oesophagus**

G06.1   Revision of interposition anastomosis of oesophagus
G06.2   Revision of anastomosis of oesophagus nec
         Includes: Revision of bypass of oesophagus nec
G06.3   Removal of bypass of oesophagus
         Includes: Conversion of interposition anastomosis to direct anastomosis of oesophagus
G06.4   Closure of bypass of oesophagus nec
G06.8   Other specified
G06.9   Unspecified
G06.0   Conversion from previous direct anastomosis of oesophagus
         Note: For use as subsiduary code when associated with construction of interposition anastomosis of oesophagus (G05)

G07   **Repair of oesophagus**

G07.1   Closure of tracheooesophageal fistula
         Includes: Excision of tracheooesophageal fistula
G07.2   Closure of fistula of oesophagus nec
         Includes: Excision of fistula of oesophagus nec
G07.3   Correction of congenital atresia of oesophagus
G07.4   Repair of rupture of oesophagus
G07.8   Other specified
G07.9   Unspecified

G08   **Artificial opening into oesophagus**

G08.1   Exteriorisation of pouch of oesophagus
G08.2   External fistulisation of oesophagus nec
G08.3   Tube oesophagostomy
         Includes: Insertion of feeding tube through artificial opening of oesophagus
G08.8   Other specified
G08.9   Unspecified
         Includes: Oesophagostomy nec

G09   **Incision of oesophagus**

G09.1   Cardiomyotomy
G09.2   Oesophagomyotomy nec
G09.3   Division of web of oesophagus
G09.4   Drainage of oesophagus
         Includes: Drainage of perioesophageal tissue
G09.8   Other specified
G09.9   Unspecified

G10   **Open operations on varices of oesophagus**
         Excludes: Portal decompression operations (L77)

G10.1   Disconnection of azygos vein
G10.2   Transection of oesophagus using staple gun
G10.3   Transection of oesophagus nec
G10.4   Local ligation of varices of oesophagus
G10.5   Open injection sclerotherapy to varices of oesophagus
G10.8   Other specified
G10.9   Unspecified

G11   **Open placement of prosthesis in oesophagus**

G11.1   Insertion of tubal prosthesis into oesophagus through stomach
G11.2   Open insertion of tubal prosthesis into oesophagus nec
G11.3   Open revision of tubal prosthesis in oesophagus
G11.4   Open removal of tubal prosthesis from oesophagus
G11.8   Other specified
G11.9   Unspecified

G13 **Other open operations on oesophagus**

G13.1 Open biopsy of lesion of oesophagus
   Includes: Open biopsy of oesophagus
G13.2 Open removal of foreign body from oesophagus
G13.8 Other specified
G13.9 Unspecified

G14 **Fibreoptic endoscopic extirpation of lesion of oesophagus**
   Excludes: When associated with general fibreoptic endoscopic examination of upper gastrointestinal tract (G45)
   Note: It is not necessary to code additionally any mention of diagnostic fibreoptic endoscopic examination limited to oesophagus (G16.9)

G14.1 Fibreoptic endoscopic snare resection of lesion of oesophagus
G14.2 Fibreoptic endoscopic laser destruction of lesion of oesophagus
G14.3 Fibreoptic endoscopic cauterisation of lesion of oesophagus
G14.4 Fibreoptic endoscopic injection sclerotherapy to varices of oesophagus
G14.5 Fibreoptic endoscopic destruction of lesion of oesophagus nec
G14.8 Other specified
G14.9 Unspecified

G15 **Other therapeutic fibreoptic endoscopic operations on oesophagus**
   Excludes: When associated with general fibreoptic endoscopic examination of upper gastrointestinal tract (G44)
   Note: It is not necessary to code additionally any mention of diagnostic fibreoptic endoscopic examination limited to oesophagus (G16.9)

G15.1 Fibreoptic endoscopic removal of foreign body from oesophagus
G15.2 Fibreoptic endoscopic balloon dilation of oesophagus
G15.3 Fibreoptic endoscopic dilation of oesophagus nec
G15.4 Fibreoptic endoscopic insertion of tubal prosthesis into oesophagus
G15.8 Other specified
G15.9 Unspecified

G16 **Diagnostic fibreoptic endoscopic examination of oesophagus**
   Excludes: When not limited to oesophagus (G45)

G16.1 Diagnostic fibreoptic endoscopic examination of oesophagus and biopsy of lesion of oesophagus
   Includes: Diagnostic fibreoptic endoscopic examination of oesophagus and biopsy of oesophagus
      Fibreoptic endoscopic biopsy of lesion of oesophagus
      Fibreoptic endoscopic biopsy of oesophagus
G16.8 Other specified
G16.9 Unspecified
   Includes: Fibreoptic oesophagoscopy nec

G17 **Endoscopic extirpation of lesion of oesophagus using rigid oesophagoscope**
   Includes: Endoscopic extirpation of lesion of stomach using rigid gastroscope
      Endoscopic extirpation of lesion of oesophagus nec
   Excludes: Endoscopic extirpation of lesion of stomach nec (G43)
   Note : It is not necessary to code additionally any mention of diagnostic endoscopic examination of oesophagus using rigid oesophagoscope (G19.9)

G17.1 Endoscopic snare resection of lesion of oesophagus using rigid oesophagoscope
G17.2 Endoscopic laser destruction of lesion of oesophagus using rigid oesophagoscope
G17.3 Endoscopic cauterisation of lesion of oesophagus using rigid oesophagoscope
G17.4 Endoscopic injection sclerotherapy to varices of oesophagus using rigid oesophagoscope
G17.8 Other specified
G17.9 Unspecified

G18   **Other therapeutic endoscopic operations on oesophagus using rigid oesophagoscope**
Includes: Therapeutic endoscopic operations on stomach using rigid gastroscope nec
            Therapeutic endoscopic operations on oesophagus nec
Excludes: Therapeutic endoscopic operations on stomach nec (G44)
Note: It is not necessary to code additionally any mention of diagnostic endoscopic examination of oesophagus using rigid oesophagoscope (G19.9)

G18.1   Endoscopic removal of foreign body from oesophagus using rigid oesophagoscope
        Includes: Removal of foreign body from oesophagus nec
G18.2   Endoscopic balloon dilation of oesophagus using rigid oesophagoscope
G18.3   Endoscopic dilation of oesophagus using rigid oesophagoscope nec
G18.4   Endoscopic insertion of tubal prosthesis into oesophagus using rigid oesophagoscope
G18.8   Other specified
G18.9   Unspecified

G19   **Diagnostic endoscopic examination of oesophagus using rigid oesophagoscope**
Includes: Diagnostic endoscopic examination of stomach using rigid gastroscope
            Diagnostic endoscopic examination of oesophagus nec
Excludes: Diagnostic endoscopic examination of stomach nec (G45)

G19.1   Diagnostic endoscopic examination of oesophagus and biopsy of lesion of oesophagus using rigid oesophagoscope
        Includes: Diagnostic endoscopic examination of oesophagus and biopsy of oesophagus using rigid oesophagoscope
            Endoscopic biopsy of lesion of oesophagus using rigid oesophagoscope
            Endoscopic biopsy of oesophagus using rigid oesophagoscope
            Biopsy of lesion of oesophagus using rigid oesophagoscope nec
            Biopsy of oesophagus using rigid oesophagoscope nec
            Biopsy of lesion of oesophagus nec
            Biopsy of oesophagus nec
        Excludes: Biopsy of lesion of stomach nec (G45.1)
            Biopsy of stomach nec (G45.1)
G19.8   Other specified
G19.9   Unspecified
        Includes: Oesophagoscopy nec

G21   **Other operations on oesophagus**

G21.1   Intubation of oesophagus for ph manometry
G21.2   Intubation of oesophagus for pressure manometry
G21.3   Intubation of oesophagus and instillation of acid or alkali hfq
G21.4   Intubation of oesophagus nec
G21.8   Other specified
G21.9   Unspecified

G23   **Repair of diaphragmatic hernia**

G23.1   Repair of oesophageal hiatus using thoracic approach
G23.2   Repair of diaphragmatic hernia using thoracic approach nec
G23.3   Repair of oesophageal hiatus using abdominal approach
G23.4   Repair of diaphragmatic hernia using abdominal approach nec
G23.8   Other specified
G23.9   Unspecified

G23   **Antireflux operations**

G24.1   Antireflux fundoplication using thoracic approach
G24.2   Antireflux operation using thoracic approach nec
G24.3   Antireflux fundoplication using abdominal approach
G24.4   Antireflux gastropexy
G24.5   Gastroplasty and antireflux procedure hfq
G24.6   Insertion of angelchick prosthesis
G24.8   Other specified
G24.9   Unspecified

G25   Revision of antireflux operations

G25.1   Revision of fundoplication of stomach
G25.2   Adjustment to angelchick prosthesis
G25.3   Removal of angelchick prosthesis
G25.8   Other specified
G25.9   Unspecified

G27   Total excision of stomach

G27.1   Total gastrectomy and excision of surrounding tissue
          Note: Use additional code as necessary for excision of lymph node (T87)
G27.2   Total gastrectomy and anastomosis of oesophagus to duodenum
G27.3   Total gastrectomy and interposition of jejunum
G27.4   Total gastrectomy and anastomosis of oesophagus to transposed jejunum
G27.5   Total gastrectomy and anastomosis of oesophagus to jejunum nec
G27.8   Other specified
G27.9   Unspecified

G28   Partial excision of stomach

G28.1   Partial gastrectomy and anastomosis of stomach to duodenum
G28.2   Partial gastrectomy and anastomosis of stomach to transposed jejunum
G28.3   Partial gastrectomy and anastomosis of stomach to jejunum nec
G28.8   Other specified
G28.9   Unspecified
          Includes: Gastrectomy nec

G29   Open extirpation of lesion of stomach

G29.1   Open excision of polyp of stomach
G29.2   Open excision of lesion of stomach nec
G29.3   Open laser destruction of lesion of stomach
G29.4   Diathermy to lesion of stomach
G29.5   Cryotherapy to lesion of stomach
G29.8   Other specified
G29.9   Unspecified

G30   Plastic operations on stomach

G30.1   Gastroplasty nec
G30.2   Partitioning of stomach
G30.8   Other specified
G30.9   Unspecified

G31   Connection of stomach to duodenum
          *Excludes: Connection of stomach to duodenum when associated with concurrent excision of stomach
                 (G27.2 G28.1)*

G31.1   Bypass of stomach by anastomosis of oesophagus to duodenum
G31.2   Bypass of stomach by anastomosis of stomach to duodenum
G31.3   Revision of anastomosis of stomach to duodenum
G31.4   Conversion to anastomosis of stomach to duodenum
          Note: Use subsidiary conversion from code as necessary
G31.8   Other specified
G31.9   Unspecified
G31.0   Conversion from previous anastomosis of stomach to duodenum

G32   **Connection of stomach to transposed jejunum**
Excludes: Connection of stomach to transposed jejunum when associated with concurrent excision of stomach (G27.4 G28.2)

G32.1   Bypass of stomach by anastomosis of stomach to transposed jejunum
G32.2   Revision of anastomosis of stomach to transposed jejunum
G32.3   Conversion to anastomosis of stomach to transposed jejunum
         Note: Use subsidiary conversion from code as necessary
G32.8   Other specified
G32.9   Unspecified
G32.0   Conversion from previous anastomosis of stomach to transposed jejunum

G33   **Other connection of stomach to jejunum**
Excludes: Connection of stomach to jejunum when associated with concurrent excision of stomach nec (G27.5 G28.3)

G33.1   Bypass of stomach by anastomosis of stomach to jejunum nec
         Includes: Gastroenterostomy nec
         Note: Use as secondary code when associated with concurrent vagotomy (A27)
G33.2   Revision of anastomosis of stomach to jejunum nec
G33.3   Conversion to anastomosis of stomach to jejunum nec
         Note: Use subsidiary conversion from code as necessary
G33.4   Open reduction of intussusception of gastroenterostomy
G33.8   Other specified
G33.9   Unspecified
G33.0   Conversion from previous anastomosis of stomach to jejunum nec

G34   **Artificial opening into stomach**

G34.1   Creation of permanent gastrostomy
G34.2   Creation of temporary gastrostomy
         Includes: Creation of gastrostomy nec
G34.3   Reconstruction of gastrostomy
G34.4   Closure of gastrostomy
G34.5   Attention to gastrostomy tube
G34.8   Other specified
G34.9   Unspecified

G35   **Operations on ulcer of stomach**

G35.1   Closure of perforated ulcer of stomach
G35.2   Closure of ulcer of stomach nec
         Includes: Suture of ulcer of stomach nec
G35.8   Other specified
G35.9   Unspecified

G36   **Other repair of stomach**

G36.1   Gastropexy nec
G36.2   Closure of perforation of stomach nec
G36.3   Closure of abnormal opening of stomach nec
G36.8   Other specified
G36.9   Unspecified

G38   **Other open operations on stomach**

G38.1   Open biopsy of lesion of stomach
         Includes: Open biopsy of stomach
G38.2   Open insertion of prosthesis into stomach
G38.3   Open insertion of feeding tube into stomach
G38.4   Open removal of foreign body from stomach
G38.5   Incision of stomach nec
         Includes: Gastrotomy nec
G38.6   Reduction of volvulus of stomach
G38.8   Other specified
G38.9   Unspecified

G40   **Incision of pylorus**

G40.1   Pyloromyotomy
          Note: *Use as secondary code when associated with concurrent vagotomy (A27)*
G40.2   Repair of congenital atresia of pylorus
G40.3   Pyloroplasty nec
          Note: *Use as secondary code when associated with concurrent vagotomy (A27)*
G40.4   Revision of pyloroplasty
G40.5   Closure of pyloroplasty
G40.6   Open dilation of pylorus
G40.8   Other specified
G40.9   Unspecified

G41   **Other operations on pylorus**

G41.1   Open biopsy of lesion of pylorus
          Includes: Open biopsy of pylorus
G41.2   Repair of perforation of pylorus
G41.8   Other specified
G41.9   Unspecified

G43   **Fibreoptic endoscopic extirpation of lesion of upper gastrointestinal tract**
          Includes: Endoscopic extirpation of lesion of upper
                      Gastrointestinal tract nec
                      Oesophagus
                      Stomach
                      Pylorus
                      Proximal duodenum
          Excludes: When associated with endoscopic examination limited to oesophagus (G14 G17)
                      When associated with endoscopic examination limited to duodenum (G54.1)
          Note: *It is not necessary to code additionally any mention of diagnostic endoscopic examination of upper gastrointestinal tract (G45.9)*
                      Use subsidiary site code as necessary

G43.1   Fibreoptic endoscopic snare resection of lesion of upper gastrointestinal tract
G43.2   Fibreoptic endoscopic laser destruction of lesion of upper gastrointestinal tract
G43.3   Fibreoptic endoscopic cauterisation of lesion of upper gastrointestinal tract
G43.4   Fibreoptic endoscopic sclerotherapy to lesion of upper gastrointestinal tract
G43.5   Fibreoptic endoscopic destruction of lesion of upper gastrointestinal tract nec
G43.8   Other specified
G43.9   Unspecified

G44   **Other fibreoptic therapeutic endoscopic operations on upper gastrointestinal tract**
          Includes: Therapeutic endoscopic operations on upper gastrointestinal tract nec
                      Oesophagus
                      Stomach
                      Pylorus
                      Proximal duodenum
          Excludes: When associated with endoscopic examination limited to oesophagus (G15 G18)
                      When associated with endoscopic examination limited to duodenum (G54)
          Note: *It is not necessary to code additionally any mention of diagnostic endoscopic examination of upper gastrointestina tract (G45.9)*
                      Use subsidiary site code as necessary

G44.1   Fibreoptic endoscopic insertion of prosthesis into upper gastrointestinal tract
G44.2   Fibreoptic endoscopic removal of foreign body from upper gastrointestinal tract
G44.3   Fibreoptic endoscopic dilation of upper gastrointestinal tract
G44.8   Other specified
G44.9   Unspecified

G45   **Diagnostic fibreoptic endoscopic examination of upper gastrointestinal tract**
Includes: Diagnostic endoscopic examination of upper gastrointestinal tract nec
           Oesophegus
           Stomach
           Pylorus
           Proximal duodenum
Excludes: When associated with examination limited to oesophagus (G16)
           When associated with examination limited to duodenum (G55)
Note: *Use subsidiary site code as necessary*

G45.1   Fibreoptic endoscopic examination of upper gastrointestinal tract and biopsy of lesion of upper gastrointestinal tract
Includes: Fibreoptic endoscopic examination of upper gastrointestinal tract and biopsy of upper gastrointestinal tract
           Fibreoptic endoscopic biopsy of lesion of upper gastrointestinal tract
           Fibreoptic endoscopic biopsy of upper gastrointestinal tract
           Biopsy of lesion of upper gastrointestinal tract nec
           Biopsy of upper gastrointestinal tract nec

G45.8   Other specified
G45.9   Unspecified
Includes: Fibreoptic gastroscopy nec
           Gastroscopy nec

G47   **Intubation of stomach**

G47.1   Intubation of stomach for ph manometry
G47.2   Intubation of stomach for pressure manometry
G47.3   Irrigation of stomach
Includes: Lavage of stomach
           Washout of stomach
G47.4   Intubation of stomach for study of gastric secretion
G47.8   Other specified
G47.9   Unspecified

G48   **Other operations on stomach**

G48.1   Insertion of gastric bubble
G48.2   Attention to gastric bubble
G48.8   Other specified
G48.9   Unspecified

G49   **Excision of duodenum**
Excludes: Pancreaticoduodenectomy (J56)

G49.1   Gastroduodenectomy

G49.2   Total excision of duodenum
G49.3   Partial excision of duodenum
G49.8   Other specified
G49.9   Unspecified
Includes: Duodenectomy nec

G50   **Open extirpation of lesion of duodenum**

G50.1   Excision of lesion of duodenum
G50.2   Open destruction of lesion of duodenum
G50.8   Other specified
G50.9   Unspecified

G51 Bypass of duodenum

G51.1 Bypass of duodenum by anastomosis of stomach to jejunum
G51.2 Bypass of duodenum by anastomosis of duodenum to duodenum
G51.3 Bypass of duodenum by anastomosis of duodenum to jejunum
G51.4 Bypass of duodenum by anastomosis of duodenum to colon
G51.8 Other specified
G51.9 Unspecified

G52 Operations on ulcer of duodenum

G52.1 Closure of perforated ulcer of duodenum
G52.2 Suture of ulcer of duodenum nec
G52.8 Other specified
G52.9 Unspecified

G53 Other open operations on duodenum

G53.1 Open biopsy of lesion of duodenum
Includes: Open biopsy of duodenum
G53.2 Closure of perforation of duodenum nec
G53.3 Open removal of foreign body from duodenum
G53.4 Open insertion of tubal prosthesis into duodenum
G53.5 Incision of duodenum nec
Includes: Duodenotomy nec
G53.6 Correction of malrotation of duodenum
G53.8 Other specified
G53.9 Unspecified

G54 Therapeutic endoscopic operations on duodenum
Excludes: When associated with general endoscopic examination of upper gastrointestinal tract (G43 G44)
When associated with endoscopic examination of biliary and pancreatic ducts (J40-J42)
Note: **It is not necessary to code additionally any mention of diagnostic endoscopic examination limited to duodenum (G55.9)**

G54.1 Endoscopic extirpation of lesion of duodenum
Includes: Snare resection of duodenum
G54.2 Endoscopic dilation of duodenum
G54.3 Endoscopic insertion of tubal prosthesis into duodenum
G54.8 Other specified
G54.9 Unspecified

G55 Diagnostic endoscopic examination of duodenum
Excludes: When not limited to duodenum (G45)

G55.1 Diagnostic endoscopic examination of duodenum and biopsy of lesion of duodenum
Includes: Diagnostic endoscopic examination of duodenum and biopsy of duodenum
Endoscopic biopsy of lesion of duodenum
Endoscopic biopsy of duodenum
Biopsy of lesion of duodenum nec
Biopsy of duodenum nec
G55.8 Other specified
G55.9 Unspecified
Includes: Duodenoscopy nec

G57 Other operations on duodenum

G57.1 Intubation of duodenum for studies of pancreatic function hfq
G57.2 Intubation of duodenum nec
G57.8 Other specified
G57.9 Unspecified

G58 Excision of jejunum

G58.1 Total jejunectomy and anastomosis of stomach to ileum
G58.2 Total jejunectomy and anastomosis of duodenum to ileum
G58.3 Total jejunectomy and anastomosis of duodenum to colon
G58.4 Partial jejunectomy and anastomosis of jejunum to ileum
Includes: Jejunectomy and anastomosis of jejunum to jejunum
G58.5 Partial jejunectomy and anastomosis of duodenum to colon
G58.8 Other specified
G58.9 Unspecified
Includes: Jejunectomy nec

G59 Extirpation of lesion of jejunum

G59.1 Excision of lesion of jejunum
G59.2 Open destruction of lesion of jejunum
G59.8 Other specified
G59.9 Unspecified

G60 Artificial opening into jejunum

G60.1 Creation of jejunostomy
G60.2 Refashioning of jejunostomy
G60.3 Closure of jejunostomy
G60.8 Other specified
G60.9 Unspecified

G61 Bypass of jejunum

G61.1 Bypass of jejunum by anastomosis of jejunum to jejunum
G61.2 Bypass of jejunum by anastomosis of jejunum to ileum
G61.3 Bypass of jejunum by anastomosis of jejunum to colon
G61.8 Other specified
G61.9 Unspecified

G62 Open endoscopic operations on jejunum

G62.1 Open jejunoscopy
Includes: Operative jejunoscopy
G62.8 Other specified
G62.9 Unspecified

G63 Other open operations on jejunum

G63.1 Open biopsy of lesion of jejunum
Includes: Open biopsy of jejunum
Biopsy of lesion of jejunum nec
Biopsy of jejunum nec
G63.2 Incision of jejunum
G63.3 Closure of perforation of jejunum
G63.4 Open intubation of jejunum
G63.8 Other specified
G63.9 Unspecified

G64 Therapeutic endoscopic operations on jejunum
Note: It is not necessary to code additionally any mention of diagnostic endoscopic examination of jejunum (G65.9)

G64.1 Endoscopic extirpation of lesion of jejunum
G64.2 Endoscopic dilation of jejunum
G64.3 Endoscopic insertion of tubal prosthesis into jejunum
G64.8 Other specified
G64.9 Unspecified

G65   **Diagnostic endoscopic examination of jejunum**

G65.1   Diagnostic endoscopic examination of jejunum and biopsy of lesion of jejunum
        Includes: Diagnostic endoscopic examination of jejunum and biopsy of jejunum
        Endoscopic biopsy of lesion of jejunum
        Endoscopic biopsy of jejunum
G65.8   Other specified
G65.9   Unspecified
        Includes: Jejunoscopy nec

G67   **Other operations on jejunum**

G67.1   Intubation of jejunum for decompression of intestine
G67.2   Intubation of jejunum for measurement of intestinal function
G67.3   Passage of crosby capsule into jejunum for biopsy of mucosa of jejunum
G67.4   Intubation of jejunum nec
G67.8   Other specified
G67.9   Unspecified

G69   **Excision of ileum**
        Includes: Small intestine nec

G69.1   Ileectomy and anastomosis of stomach to ileum
G69.2   Ileectomy and anastomosis of duodenum to ileum
G69.3   Ileectomy and anastomosis of ileum to ileum
G69.4   Ileectomy and anastomosis of ileum to colon
G69.8   Other specified
G69.9   Unspecified
        Includes: Ileectomy nec

G70   **Open extirpation of lesion of ileum**
        Includes: Small intestine nec

G70.1   Excision of meckel diverticulum
G70.2   Excision of lesion of ileum nec
G70.3   Open destruction of lesion of ileum
G70.8   Other specified
G70.9   Unspecified

G71   **Bypass of ileum**
        Includes: Small intestine nec

G71.1   Bypass of ileum by anastomosis of jejunum to ileum
G71.2   Bypass of ileum by anastomosis of ileum to ileum
G71.3   Bypass of ileum by anastomosis of ileum to caecum
G71.4   Bypass of ileum by anastomosis of ileum to transverse colon
G71.5   Bypass of ileum by anastomosis of ileum to colon nec
        Includes: Bypass of ileum by anastomosis of ileum to rectum
G71.8   Other specified
G71.9   Unspecified

G72   **Other connection of ileum**
        Includes: Small intestine nec
        Excludes: When associated with concurrent excision of ileum (G69)

G72.1   Anastomosis of ileum to caecum
G72.2   Anastomosis of ileum to transverse colon
G72.3   Anastomosis of ileum to colon nec
G72.4   Anastomosis of ileum to rectum
G72.5   Anastomosis of ileum to anus and creation of pouch hfq
G72.8   Other specified
G72.9   Unspecified

G73   **Attention to connection of ileum**
Includes: Small intestine nec

G73.1   Revision of anastomosis of ileum
G73.2   Closure of anastomosis of ileum
G73.8   Other specified
G73.9   Unspecified

G74   **Creation of artificial opening into ileum**
Includes: Small intestine nec

G74.1   Creation of continent ileostomy
G74.2   Creation of temporary ileostomy
G74.3   Creation of defunctioning ileostomy
         Includes: Creation of split ileostomy
G74.8   Other specified
G74.9   Unspecified

G75   **Attention to artificial opening into ileum**
Includes: Small intestine nec

G75.1   Refashioning of ileostomy
G75.2   Repair of prolapse of ileostomy
G75.3   Closure of ileostomy
G75.4   Dilation of ileostomy
G75.5   Reduction of prolapse of ileostomy
G75.8   Other specified
G75.9   Unspecified

G76   **Intraabdominal manipulation of ileum**
Includes: Small intestine nec

G76.1   Open reduction of intussusception of ileum
G76.2   Open relief of strangulation of ileum
G76.3   Open relief of obstruction of ileum nec
G76.4   Plication of ileum
G76.8   Other specified
G76.9   Unspecified

G78   **Other open operations on ileum**
Includes: Small intestine nec

G78.1   Open biopsy of lesion of ileum
         Includes: Open biopsy of ileum
                    Biopsy of lesion of ileum nec
                    Biopsy of ileum nec
G78.2   Strictureplasty of ileum
G78.3   Removal of foreign body from ileum
G78.4   Closure of perforation of ileum
G78.5   Exclusion of segment of ileum
G78.6   Open intubation of ileum
G78.8   Other specified
G78.9   Unspecified

G79   **Therapeutic endoscopic operations on ileum**
Includes: Small intestine nec
Note: *It is not necessary to code additionally any mention of diagnostic endoscopic examination of ileum (G80.9)*

G79.1   Endoscopic extirpation of lesion of ileum
G79.2   Endoscopic dilation of ileum
G79.3   Endoscopic insertion of tubal prosthesis into ileum
G79.8   Other specified
G79.9   Unspecified

G80   **Diagnostic endoscopic examination of ileum**
Includes: Small intestine nec

G80.1   Diagnostic endoscopic examination of ileum and biopsy of lesion of ileum
Includes: Diagnostic endoscopic examination of ileum and biopsy of ileum
Endoscopic biopsy of lesion of ileum
Endoscopic biopsy of ileum

G80.8   Other specified
G80.9   Unspecified
Includes: Ileoscopy nec
Enteroscopy nec

G82   **Other operations on ileum**
Includes: Small intestine nec

G82.1   Radiological reduction of intussusception of ileum using barium enema
G82.2   Intubation of ileum for decompression of intestine
G82.3   Intubation of ileum for studies on function hfq
G82.4   Intubation of ileum nec
G82.8   Other specified
G82.9   Unspecified

CHAPTER H

LOWER DIGESTIVE TRACT

(CODES H01-H62)

H01   Emergency excision of appendix

H01.1   Emergency excision of abnormal appendix and drainage hfq
H01.2   Emergency excision of abnormal appendix nec
H01.3   Emergency excision of normal appendix
H01.8   Other specified
H01.9   Unspecified
         Includes: Emergency appendicectomy nec

H02   Other excision of appendix

H02.1   Interval appendicectomy
H02.2   Planned delayed appendicectomy nec
H02.3   Prophylactic appendicectomy nec
H02.4   Incidental appendicectomy
         Includes: Appendicectomy performed during course of other abdominal operation
         Note: Use as secondary code when performed during creation of caecostomy (H14.9)
H02.8   Other specified
H02.9   Unspecified
         Includes: Appendicectomy nec

H03   Other operations on appendix

H03.1   Drainage of abscess of appendix
H03.2   Drainage of appendix nec
H03.8   Other specified
H03.9   Unspecified

H04   Total excision of colon and rectum

H04.1   Panproctocolectomy and ileostomy
         Includes: Proctocolectomy nec
H04.2   Panproctocolectomy and anastomosis of ileum to anus and creation of pouch hfq
H04.3   Panproctocolectomy and anastomosis of ileum to anus nec
H04.8   Other specified
H04.9   Unspecified

H05   Total excision of colon

H05.1   Total colectomy and anastomosis of ileum to rectum
H05.2   Total colectomy and ileostomy and creation of rectal fistula hfq
H05.3   Total colectomy and ileostomy nec
H05.8   Other specified
H05.9   Unspecified

H06   Extended excision of right hemicolon
         Includes: Excision of right colon and other segment of ileum or colon and surrounding tissue
                   Caecum

H06.1   Extended right hemicolectomy and end to end anastomosis
H06.2   Extended right hemicolectomy and anastomosis of ileum to colon
H06.3   Extended right hemicolectomy and anastomosis nec
H06.4   Extended right hemicolectomy and ileostomy hfq
H06.8   Other specified
H06.9   Unspecified

H07   **Other excision of right hemicolon**
Includes: Limited excision of caecum and terminal ileum caecum

H07.1   Right hemicolectomy and end to end anastomosis of ileum to colon
Includes: Ileocaecal resection
H07.2   Right hemicolectomy and side to side anastomosis of ileum to transverse colon
H07.3   Right hemicolectomy and anastomosis nec
H07.4   Right hemicolectomy and ileostomy hfq
H07.8   Other specified
H07.9   Unspecified

H08   **Excision of transverse colon**

H08.1   Transverse colectomy and end to end anastomosis
H08.2   Transverse colectomy and anastomosis of ileum to colon
H08.3   Transverse colectomy and anastomosis nec
H08.4   Transverse colectomy and ileostomy hfq
H08.5   Transverse colectomy and exteriorisation of bowel nec
Note: Use secondary code for type of exteriorisation of bowel (H14 H15)
H08.8   Other specified
H08.9   Unspecified

H09   **Excision of left hemicolon**

H09.1   Left hemicolectomy and end to end anastomosis of colon to rectum
H09.2   Left hemicolectomy and end to end anastomosis of colon to colon
H09.3   Left hemicolectomy and anastomosis nec
H09.4   Left hemicolectomy and ileostomy hfq
H09.5   Left hemicolectomy and exteriorisation of bowel nec
Note: Use secondary code for type of exteriorisation of bowel (H14 H15)
H09.8   Other specified
H09.9   Unspecified

H10   **Excision of sigmoid colon**

H10.1   Sigmoid colectomy and end to end anastomosis of ileum to rectum
H10.2   Sigmoid colectomy and anastomosis of colon to rectum
H10.3   Sigmoid colectomy and anastomosis nec
H10.4   Sigmoid colectomy and ileostomy hfq
H10.5   Sigmoid colectomy and exteriorisation of bowel nec
Note: Use secondary code for type of exteriorisation of bowel (H14 H15)
H10.8   Other specified
H10.9   Unspecified

H11   **Other excision of colon**
Includes: Excision of colon where segment removed is not stated

H11.1   Colectomy and end to end anastomosis of colon to colon nec
H11.2   Colectomy and side to side anastomosis of ileum to colon nec
H11.3   Colectomy and anastomosis nec
H11.4   Colectomy and ileostomy nec
H11.5   Colectomy and exteriorisation of bowel nec
Note: Use secondary code for type of exteriorisation of bowel (H14 H15)
H11.8   Other specified
H11.9   Unspecified
Includes: Colectomy nec
Hemicolectomy nec

H12   **Extirpation of lesion of colon**
Includes: Caecum

H12.1   Excision of diverticulum of colon
H12.2   Excision of lesion of colon nec
H12.3   Destruction of lesion of colon nec
H12.8   Other specified
H12.9   Unspecified

H13 **Bypass of colon**
Includes: Caecum
Excludes: Bypass of colon when associated with excision of colon (H04-H11)

H13.1 Bypass of colon by anastomosis of ileum to colon
H13.2 Bypass of colon by anastomosis of caecum to sigmoid colon
H13.3 Bypass of colon by anastomosis of transverse colon to sigmoid colon
H13.4 Bypass of colon by anastomosis of transverse colon to rectum
H13.5 Bypass of colon by anastomosis of colon to rectum nec
H13.8 Other specified
H13.9 Unspecified

H14 **Exteriorisation of caecum**

H14.1 Tube caecostomy
H14.2 Refashioning of caecostomy
H14.3 Closure of caecostomy
H14.8 Other specified
H14.9 Unspecified
Includes: Caecostomy nec

H15 **Other exteriorisation of colon**

H15.1 Loop colostomy
H15.2 End colostomy
H15.3 Refashioning of colostomy
H15.4 Closure of colostomy
H15.5 Dilation of colostomy
H15.6 Reduction of prolapse of colostomy
H15.8 Other specified
H15.9 Unspecified
Includes: Colostomy nec

H16 **Incision of colon**
Includes: Caecum

H16.1 Drainage of colon
Includes: Drainage of pericolonic tissue
H16.2 Caecotomy
H16.3 Colotomy
H16.8 Other specified
H16.9 Unspecified

H17 **Intraabdominal manipulation of colon**
Includes: Caecum

H17.1 Open reduction of intussusception of colon
H17.2 Open reduction of volvulus of caecum
H17.3 Open reduction of volvulus of sigmoid colon
H17.4 Open reduction of volvulus of colon nec
H17.5 Open relief of strangulation of colon
H17.6 Open relief of obstruction of colon nec
H17.8 Other specified
H17.9 Unspecified

H18 **Open endoscopic operations on colon**
Includes: Caecum

H18.1 Open colonoscopy
Includes: Operative colonoscopy
H18.8 Other specified
H18.9 Unspecified

H19   **Other open operations on colon**
Includes: Caecum
Excludes: Repair of intestinovesical fistula (M37.2)

H19.1   Open biopsy of lesion of colon
Includes: Open biopsy of colon
Biopsy of lesion of colon
Biopsy of colon
H19.2   Fixation of colon
H19.3   Enterorrhaphy of colon
H19.4   Open removal of foreign body from colon
H19.8   Other specified
H19.9   Unspecified

H20   **Endoscopic extirpation of lesion of colon**
Includes: Caecum
Mucosa of colon
Mucosa of caecum
Excludes: Fibreoptic endoscopic extirpation of lesion limited to sigmoid colon (H23)
Note: It is not necessary to code additionally any mention of diagnostic endoscopic examination limited to colon (H22.9)
Use subsidiary site code as necessary

H20.1   Fibreoptic endoscopic snare resection of lesion of colon
H20.2   Fibreoptic endoscopic cauterisation of lesion of colon
H20.3   Fibreoptic endoscopic laser destruction of lesion of colon
H20.4   Fibreoptic endoscopic destruction of lesion of colon nec
H20.8   Other specified
H20.9   Unspecified

H21   **Other therapeutic endoscopic operations on colon**
Includes: Caecum
Mucosa of colon
Mucosa of caecum
Excludes: Other therapeutic fibreoptic endoscopic operations limited to sigmoid colon (H24)
Note: It is not necessary to code additionally any mention of diagnostic endoscopic examination limited to on (H22.9)
Use subsidiary site code as necessary

H21.1   Fibreoptic endoscopic dilation of colon
H21.2   Fibreoptic endoscopic coagulation of blood vessel of colon
H21.3   Fibreoptic endoscopic removal of foreign body from colon
H21.8   Other specified
H21.9   Unspecified

H22   **Diagnostic endoscopic examination of colon**
Includes: Caecum
Mucosa of colon
Mucosa of caecum
Excludes: Diagnostic fibreoptic endoscopic examination limited to sigmoid colon (H25)
Note: Use subsidiary site code as necessary

H22.1   Diagnostic fibreoptic endoscopic examination of colon and biopsy of lesion of colon
Includes: Diagnostic fibreoptic endoscopic examination of colon and biopsy of colon
Fibreoptic endoscopic biopsy of lesion of colon
Fibreoptic endoscopic biopsy of colon
H22.8   Other specified
H22.9   Unspecified
Includes: Colonoscopy nec

H23   **Endoscopic extirpation of lesion of lower bowel using fibreoptic sigmoidoscope**
Includes: Sigmoid colon
Colon
Rectum
Note: *It is not necessary to code additionally any mention of diagnostic endoscopic examination of
lower bowel using fibreoptic sigmoidoscope (H25.9)*
Use subsidiary site code as necessary

H23.1   Endoscopic snare resection of lesion of lower bowel using fibreoptic sigmoidoscope
H23.2   Endoscopic cauterisation of lesion of lower bowel using fibreoptic sigmoidoscope
H23.3   Endoscopic laser destruction of lesion of lower bowel using fibreoptic sigmoidoscope
H23.4   Endoscopic destruction of lesion of lower bowel using fibreoptic sigmoidoscope nec
H23.8   Other specified
H23.9   Unspecified

H24   **Other therapeutic endoscopic operations on lower bowel using fibreoptic sigmoidoscope**
Includes: Sigmoid colon
Colon
Rectum
Note: *It is not necessary to code additionally any mention of diagnostic endoscopic examination of
lower bowel using fibreoptic sigmoidoscope (H25.9)*
Use subsidiary site code as necessary

H24.1   Endoscopic dilation of lower bowel using fibreoptic sigmoidoscope
H24.2   Endoscopic coagulation of blood vessel of lower bowel using fibreoptic sigmoidoscope
H24.3   Endoscopic insertion of tubal prosthesis into lower bowel using fibreoptic sigmoidoscope
H24.8   Other specified
H24.9   Unspecified

H25   **Diagnostic endoscopic examination of lower bowel using fibreoptic sigmoidoscope**
Includes: Sigmoid colon
Colon
Rectum
Excludes: General diagnostic examination of colon (H22.9)
Note: *Use subsidiary site code as necessary*

H25.1   Diagnostic endoscopic examination of lower bowel and biopsy of lesion of lower bowel using fibreoptic
sigmoidoscope
*Includes: Diagnostic endoscopic examination of lower bowel and biopsy of lower bowel using fibreoptic
sigmoidoscope*
Endoscopic biopsy of lesion of lower bowel using fibreoptic sigmoidoscope
Endoscopic biopsy of lower bowel using fibreoptic sigmoidoscope
H25.8   Other specified
H25.9   Unspecified
Includes: Fibreoptic sigmoidoscopy nec
Fibrosigmoidoscopy nec

H26   **Endoscopic extirpation of lesion of sigmoid colon using rigid sigmoidoscope**
Includes: Endoscopic extirpation of lesion of sigmoid colon nec
Rectum
Note: *It is not necessary to code additionally any mention of diagnostic endoscopic operations on
sigmoid colon using rigid sigmoidoscope (H28.9)*
Use subsidiary site code as necessary

H26.1   Endoscopic snare resection of lesion of sigmoid colon using rigid sigmoidoscope
H26.2   Endoscopic cauterisation of lesion of sigmoid colon using rigid sigmoidoscope
H26.3   Endoscopic laser destruction of lesion of sigmoid colon using rigid sigmoidoscope
H26.4   Endoscopic cryotherapy to lesion of sigmoid colon using rigid sigmoidoscope
H26.5   Endoscopic destruction of lesion of sigmoid colon using rigid sigmoidoscope nec
H26.8   Other specified
H26.9   Unspecified

H27 **Other therapeutic endoscopic operations on sigmoid colon using rigid sigmoidoscope**
Includes: Endoscopic operations on sigmoid colon nec
Rectum
Note: **It is not necessary to code additionally any mention of diagnostic endoscopic examination of sigmoid colon using rigid sigmoidoscope (H28.9)**
Use subsidiary site code as necessary

H27.1 Endoscopic dilation of sigmoid colon using rigid sigmoidoscope
H27.2 Endoscopic removal of foreign body from sigmoid colon using rigid sigmoidoscope
H27.3 Endoscopic insertion of tubal prosthesis into sigmoid colon using rigid sigmoidoscope
H27.8 Other specified
H27.9 Unspecified

H28 **Diagnostic endoscopic examination of sigmoid colon using rigid sigmoidoscope**
Includes: Diagnostic endoscopic examination of sigmoid colon nec
Rectum
Note: **Use subsidiary site code as necessary**

H28.1 Diagnostic endoscopic examination of sigmoid colon and biopsy of lesion of sigmoid colon using rigid sigmoidoscope
Includes: Diagnostic endoscopic examination of sigmoid colon and biopsy of sigmoid colon using rigid sigmoidoscope
Endoscopic biopsy of lesion of lower bowel using rigid sigmoidoscope
Endoscopic biopsy of lower bowel using rigid sigmoidoscope
Biopsy of lesion of sigmoid colon using rigid sigmoidoscope
Biopsy of sigmoid colon using rigid sigmoidoscope
H28.8 Other specified
H28.9 Unspecified
Includes: Sigmoidoscopy nec

H30 **Other operations on colon**

H30.1 Radiological reduction of intussusception of colon using barium enema
H30.2 Intubation of colon for pressure manometry
H30.3 Passage of flatus tube to reduce volvulus of sigmoid colon
H30.4 Intubation of colon nec
H30.5 Irrigation of colon
Includes: Lavage of colon
Washout of colon
H30.8 Other specified
H30.9 Unspecified

H33 **Excision of rectum**
Includes: Excision of whole or part of rectum with or without part of sigmoid colon

H33.1 Abdominoperineal excision of rectum and end colostomy
H33.2 Proctectomy and anastomosis of colon to anus
H33.3 Anterior resection of rectum and anastomosis of colon to rectum using staples
Includes: Rectosigmoidectomy and anastomosis of colon to rectum
H33.4 Anterior resection of rectum and anastomosis nec
H33.5 Rectosigmoidectomy and closure of rectal stump and exteriorisation of bowel
Note: *Use secondary code for type of exteriorisation of bowel (G74 H14-H15)*
H33.6 Anterior resection of rectum and exteriorisation of bowel
Note: *Use secondary code for type of exteriorisation of bowel (G74 H14-H15)*
H33.8 Other specified
H33.9 Unspecified
Includes: Rectosigmoidectomy nec

H34 **Open extirpation of lesion of rectum**

H34.1 Open excision of lesion of rectum
H34.2 Open cauterisation of lesion of rectum
H34.3 Open cryotherapy to lesion of rectum
H34.4 Open laser destruction of lesion of rectum
H34.5 Open destruction of lesion of rectum nec
H34.8 Other specified
H34.9 Unspecified

H35 **Fixation of rectum for prolapse**

H35.1 Anterior fixation of rectum
H35.2 Posterior fixation of rectum using prosthetic material
H35.3 Posterior fixation of rectum nec
H35.4 Fixation of rectum using fascia lata
H35.8 Other specified
H35.9 Unspecified

H36 **Other abdominal operations for prolapse of rectum**

H36.1 Abdominal repair of levator ani muscles
       Includes: Repair of levator ani muscles nec
                 Repair of pelvic floor muscles nec
H36.8 Other specified
H36.9 Unspecified

H40 **Operations on rectum through anal sphincter**

H40.1 Transsphincteric excision of mucosa of rectum
H40.2 Transsphincteric excision of lesion of rectum
       Includes: Transsphincteric biopsy of lesion of rectum
                 Transsphincteric biopsy of rectum
H40.3 Transsphincteric destruction of lesion of rectum
H40.4 Transsphincteric anastomosis of colon to anus
H40.8 Other specified
H40.9 Unspecified

H41 **Other operations on rectum through anus**

H41.1 Rectosigmoidectomy and peranal anastomosis
H41.2 Peranal excision of lesion of rectum
       Includes: Peranal biopsy of lesion of rectum
                 Peranal biopsy of rectum
H41.3 Peranal destruction of lesion of rectum
H41.4 Peranal mucosal proctectomy and endoanal anastomosis
H41.8 Other specified
H41.9 Unspecified

H42 **Perineal operations for prolapse of rectum**
       Includes: Perineal operations for prolapse of mucosa of rectum

H42.1 Insertion of encircling suture around perianal sphincter
       Includes: Insertion of thiersch wire around perianal sphincter
                 Insertion of suture around perianal sphincter
H42.2 Perineal plication of levator ani muscles and anal sphincters
H42.3 Insertion of supralevator sling
H42.4 Removal of encircling suture from around perianal sphincter
H42.5 Excision of mucosal prolapse of rectum nec
H42.6 Perineal repair of prolapse of rectum nec
H42.8 Other specified
H42.9 Unspecified

H44 Manipulation of rectum

H44.1 Manual removal of foreign body from rectum
H44.2 Manual reduction of prolapse of rectum
H44.3 Manual evacuation of impacted faeces from rectum
H44.4 Examination of rectum under anaesthetic
H44.5 Massage of rectum
H44.8 Other specified
H44.9 Unspecified

H46 Other operations on rectum

H46.1 Radiological reduction of intussusception of rectum using barium enema
H46.2 Hydrostatic reduction of intussusception of rectum
H46.3 Intubation of rectum for pressure manometry
H46.4 Intubation of rectum nec
H46.8 Other specified
H46.9 Unspecified

H47 Excision of anus

H47.1 Excision of sphincter of anus
H47.8 Other specified
H47.9 Unspecified

H48 Excision of lesion of anus
Includes: Perianal region

H48.1 Excision of polyp of anus
H48.2 Excision of skin tag of anus
H48.3 Excision of perianal wart
H48.8 Other specified
H48.9 Unspecified

H49 Destruction of lesion of anus
Includes: Perianal region

H49.1 Cauterisation of lesion of anus
H49.2 Laser destruction of lesion of anus
H49.3 Cryotherapy to lesion of anus
H49.8 Other specified
H49.9 Unspecified

H50 Repair of anus

H50.1 Posterior repair of anal sphincter
H50.2 Anterior repair of anal sphincter
H50.3 Cutback of covered anus
H50.4 Reanastomosis of rectum to anal canal for correction of congenital atresia of rectum
H50.8 Other specified
H50.9 Unspecified
Includes: Anoplasty nec

H51 Excision of haemorrhoid

H51.1 Haemorrhoidectomy
Includes: Formal haemorrhoidectomy
H51.2 Partial internal sphincterotomy for haemorrhoid
H51.8 Other specified
H51.9 Unspecified

H52   **Destruction of haemorrhoid**

H52.1   Cryotherapy to haemorrhoid
H52.2   Infra red photocoagulation of haemorrhoid
H52.3   Injection of sclerosing substance into haemorrhoid
         Includes: Injection into haemorrhoid
                   Sclerotherapy to haemorrhoid
H52.4   Rubber band ligation of haemorrhoid
H52.8   Other specified
H52.9   Unspecified

H53   **Other operations on haemorrhoid**

H53.1   Evacuation of perianal haematoma
         Includes: Evacuation of thrombosed haemorrhoid
H53.2   Forced manual dilation of anus for haemorrhoid
H53.3   Manual reduction of prolapsed haemorrhoid
H53.8   Other specified
H53.9   Unspecified

H54   **Dilation of anal sphincter**

H54.1   Anorectal stretch
         Excludes: Forced manual dilation for haemorrhoid (H53.2)
H54.8   Other specified
H54.9   Unspecified

H55   **Other operations on perianal region**

H55.1   Laying open of low anal fistula
H55.2   Laying open of high anal fistula
H55.3   Laying open of anal fistula nec
H55.4   Insertion of seton into high anal fistula and partial laying open of track hfq
H55.5   Fistulography of anal fistula
H55.8   Other specified
H55.9   Unspecified

H56   **Other operations on anus**

H56.1   Biopsy of lesion of anus
         Includes: Biopsy of anus
H56.2   Lateral sphincterotomy of anus
H56.3   Incision of septum of anus
H56.4   Excision of anal fissure
H56.8   Other specified
H56.9   Unspecified

H58   **Drainage through perineal region**

H58.1   Drainage of ischiorectal abscess
H58.2   Drainage of perianal abscess
H58.3   Drainage of perirectal abscess
H58.8   Other specified
H58.9   Unspecified

H59   **Excision of pilonidal sinus**

H59.1   Excision of pilonidal sinus and Z plasty skin flap hfq
H59.2   Excision of pilonidal sinus and skin flap nec
H59.3   Excision of pilonidal sinus and skin graft hfq
H59.4   Excision of pilonidal sinus and suture hfq
H59.8   Other specified
H59.9   Unspecified

H60   **Other operations on pilonidal sinus**

H60.1   Destruction of pilonidal sinus
H60.2   Laying open of pilonidal sinus
H60.3   Drainage of pilonidal sinus
H60.4   Injection of radiocontrast substance into pilonidal sinus
      Includes: Sinography of pilonidal sinus
H60.8   Other specified
H60.9   Unspecified

H62   **Other operations on bowel**
      Includes: Sigmoid colon
               Colon
               Rectum

H62.1   Laser recanalisation of bowel nec
H62.2   Mobilisation of bowel nec
H62.3   Dilation of bowel nec
H62.4   Intubation of bowel nec
H62.5   Irrigation of bowel nec
      Includes: Lavage of bowel nec
               Washout of bowel nec
H62.8   Other specified
H62.9   Unspecified

CHAPTER J

OTHER ABDOMINAL ORGANS - PRINCIPALLY DIGESTIVE

(CODES J01-J72)

J01   **Transplantation of liver**

J01.1   Orthotopic transplantation of liver
J01.2   Heterotopic transplantation of liver
        Includes: Piggy back transplantation of liver
        Auxillary transplantation of liver
J01.3   Replacement of previous liver transplant
J01.8   Other specified
J01.9   Unspecified

J02   **Partial excision of liver**

J02.1   Right hemihepatectomy
J02.2   Left hemihepatectomy
J02.3   Resection of segment of liver
J02.4   Wedge excision of liver
J02.5   Marsupialisation of lesion of liver
J02.8   Other specified
J02.9   Unspecified

J03   **Extirpation of lesion of liver**

J03.1   Excision of lesion of liver
J03.2   Destruction of lesion of liver
J03.8   Other specified
J03.9   Unspecified

J04   **Repair of liver**

J04.1   Removal of lacerated fragment of liver
J04.2   Repair of laceration of liver
J04.3   Packing of laceration of liver
J04.8   Other specified
J04.9   Unspecified

J05   **Incision of liver**

J05.1   Open drainage of liver
J05.2   Open removal of calculus from liver
J05.3   Open wedge biopsy of lesion of liver
        Includes: Open wedge biopsy of liver
        Open biopsy of lesion of liver
        Open biopsy of liver
J05.8   Other specified
J05.9   Unspecified

J07   **Other open operations on liver**

J07.1   Open devascularisation of liver
J07.2   Open insertion of cannula for perfusion of liver
J07.3   Exploration of liver
J07.8   Other specified
J07.9   Unspecified

J08 **Therapeutic endoscopic operations on liver using laparoscope**
Includes: Therapeutic endoscopic operations on liver using peritoneoscope
Therapeutic endoscopic operations on liver
Gall bladder
Excludes: When associated with general examination of peritoneum (T42)
Note: ***It is not necessary to code additionally any mention of diagnostic endoscopic examination of liver using laparoscope (J09.9)***

J08.1 Endoscopic removal of calculus from liver using laparoscope
J08.2 Endoscopic insertion of cannula into gall bladder using laparoscope
J08.8 Other specified
J08.9 Unspecified

J09 **Diagnostic endoscopic examination of liver using laparoscope**
Includes: Diagnostic endoscopic examination of liver using peritoneoscope
Diagnostic endoscopic examination of liver
Gall bladder
Excludes: Diagnostic endoscopic examination of liver using laparoscope when associated with general examination of the peritoneum (T43)

J09.1 Diagnostic endoscopic examination of liver and biopsy of lesion of liver using laparoscope
Includes: Diagnostic endoscopic examination of liver and biopsy of liver using laparoscope
Endoscopic biopsy of lesion of liver using laparoscope
Endoscopic biopsy of liver using laparoscope
J09.8 Other specified
J09.9 Unspecified

J10 **Transluminal operations on blood vessel of liver**
Note: Use subsidiary code to identify method of image control as necessary (Y53)

J10.1 Percutaneous transluminal embolisation of hepatic artery
J10.2 Percutaneous transluminal embolisation of portal vein
J10.3 Percutaneous transluminal injection of therapeutic substance into liver
J10.8 Other specified
J10.9 Unspecified

J12 **Other therapeutic percutaneous operations on liver**
Note: Use subsidiary code to identify method of image control as necessary (Y53)

J12.1 Percutaneous drainage of liver
J12.2 Percutaneous removal of calculus from liver
J12.8 Other specified
J12.9 Unspecified

J13 **Diagnostic percutaneous operations on liver**
Note: Use subsidiary code to identify method of image control as necessary (Y53)

J13.1 Percutaneous transvascular biopsy of lesion of liver
Includes: Percutaneous transluminal biopsy of lesion of liver
Percutaneous transluminal biopsy of liver
Transjugular biopsy of lesion of liver
Transjugular biopsy of liver
J13.2 Percutaneous biopsy of lesion of liver nec
Includes: Percutaneous biopsy of liver nec
J13.8 Other specified
J13.9 Unspecified

J14 **Other puncture of liver**
Excludes: Under image control (J10-J13)

J14.1 Biopsy of liver nec
Includes: Biopsy of lesion of liver nec
J14.2 Aspiration of liver nec
J14.8 Other specified
J14.9 Unspecified

J16   Other operations on liver

J16.1   Localised perfusion of liver
J16.2   Extracorporeal assistance to liver
J16.8   Other specified
J16.9   Unspecified

J18   Excision of gall bladder

J18.1   Total cholecystectomy and excision of surrounding tissue
J18.2   Total cholecystectomy and exploration of common bile duct
         Includes: Cholecystectomy and exploration of common bile duct nec
J18.3   Total cholecystectomy nec
         Includes: Cholecystectomy nec
J18.4   Partial cholecystectomy and exploration of common bile duct
J18.5   Partial cholecystectomy nec
J18.8   Other specified
J18.9   Unspecified

J19   Connection of gall bladder

J19.1   Anastomosis of gall bladder to stomach
J19.2   Anastomosis of gall bladder to duodenum
J19.3   Anastomosis of gall bladder to jejunum
J19.4   Anastomosis of gall bladder to intestine nec
J19.5   Revision of anastomosis of gall bladder
J19.6   Closure of anastomosis of gall bladder
J19.8   Other specified
J19.9   Unspecified

J20   Repair of gall bladder

J20.1   Closure of fistula of gall bladder
J20.2   Closure of cholecystotomy
J20.3   Repair of perforation of gall bladder
J20.8   Other specified
J20.9   Unspecified

J21   Incision of gall bladder

J21.1   Open removal of calculus from gall bladder
J21.2   Drainage of gall bladder
         Includes: Cholecystostomy nec
J21.3   Drainage of tissue surrounding gall bladder
J21.8   Other specified
J21.9   Unspecified

J23   Other open operations on gall bladder

J23.1   Excision of lesion of gall bladder
J23.2   Open biopsy of lesion of gall bladder
         Includes: Open biopsy of gall bladder
                    Biopsy of lesion of gall bladder nec
                    Biopsy of gall bladder nec
J23.3   Exploration of gall bladder
J23.8   Other specified
J23.9   Unspecified

J24　**Therapeutic percutaneous operations on gall bladder**
　　　　Note:　Use subsidiary code to identify method of image control as necessary (Y53)

J24.1　Percutaneous drainage of gall bladder
J24.2　Percutaneous fragmentation of calculus in gall bladder
　　　　Includes: Percutaneous lithotripsy of calculus in gall bladder
J24.3　Percutaneous dissolution therapy to calculus in gall bladder
J24.8　Other specified
J24.9　Unspecified

J25　**Diagnostic percutaneous operations on gall bladder**
　　　　Note:　Use subsidiary code to identify method of image control as necessary (Y53)

J25.1　Percutaneous biopsy of lesion of gall bladder
　　　　Includes: Percutaneous biopsy of gall bladder
J25.8　Other specified
J25.9　Unspecified

J26　**Other operations on gall bladder**

J26.1　Extracorporeal fragmentation of calculus in gall bladder
　　　　Includes: Extracorporeal lithotripsy of calculus in gall bladder
J26.8　Other specified
J26.9　Unspecified

J27　**Excision of bile duct**

J27.1　Excision of ampulla of vater and replantation of common bile duct into duodenum
J27.2　Partial excision of bile duct and anastomosis of bile duct to duodenum
J27.3　Partial excision of bile duct and anastomosis of bile duct to jejunum
J27.4　Partial excision of bile duct and end to end anastomosis of bile duct
J27.8　Other specified
J27.9　Unspecified

J28　**Extirpation of lesion of bile duct**

J28.1　Excision of lesion of bile duct
J28.2　Destruction of lesion of bile duct
J28.8　Other specified
J28.9　Unspecified

J29　**Connection of hepatic duct**

J29.1　Anastomosis of hepatic duct to transposed jejunum and insertion of tubal prosthesis hfq
J29.2　Anastomosis of hepatic duct to jejunum nec
J29.3　Revision of anastomosis of hepatic duct
J29.4　Open dilation of anastomosis of hepatic duct
J29.8　Other specified
J29.9　Unspecified

J30　**Connection of common bile duct**

J30.1　Anastomosis of common bile duct to duodenum
J30.2　Anastomosis of common bile duct to transposed jejunum
J30.3　Anastomosis of common bile duct to jejunum nec
J30.4　Revision of anastomosis of common bile duct
J30.5　Open dilation of anastomosis of common bile duct
J30.8　Other specified
J30.9　Unspecified

J31   **Open introduction of prosthesis into bile duct**

J31.1   Open insertion of tubal prosthesis into both hepatic ducts and common bile duct
J31.2   Open insertion of tubal prosthesis into one hepatic duct and common bile duct
J31.3   Open renewal of tubal prosthesis in bile duct
J31.4   Open removal of tubal prosthesis from bile duct
J31.8   Other specified
J31.9   Unspecified

J32   **Repair of bile duct**

J32.1   Reconstruction of bile duct
J32.2   Reanastomosis of bile duct
          Includes: End to end anastomosis of divided bile duct
J32.8   Other specified
J32.9   Unspecified

J33   **Incision of bile duct**

J33.1   Open removal of calculus from bile duct and drainage of bile duct
J33.2   Open removal of calculus from bile duct nec
J33.3   Drainage of bile duct nec
J33.8   Other specified
J33.9   Unspecified
          Includes: Exploration of bile duct
          Excludes: Exploration of bile duct when associated with excision of gall bladder (J18)

J34   **Plastic repair of sphincter of Oddi using duodenal approach**
          Includes: Plastic repair of sphincter of Oddi nec

J34.1   Sphincteroplasty of bile duct and pancreatic duct using duodenal approach
J34.2   Sphincteroplasty of bile duct using duodenal approach nec
J34.3   Sphincteroplasty of pancreatic duct using duodenal approach nec
J34.8   Other specified
J34.9   Unspecified
          Includes: Sphincteroplasty of papilla of Vater using duodenal approach
          *   Sphincteroplasty of papilla of Vater nec*

J35   **Incision of sphincter of Oddi using duodenal approach**
          Includes: Incision of sphincter of Oddi nec

J35.1   Sphincterotomy of bile duct and pancreatic duct using duodenal approach
J35.2   Sphincterotomy of bile duct using duodenal approach nec
J35.3   Sphincterotomy of pancreatic duct using duodenal approach nec
J35.8   Other specified
J35.9   Unspecified
          Includes: Sphincterotomy of papilla of Vater using duodenal approach
          *   Sphincterotomy of papilla of Vater nec*

J36   **Other operations on ampulla of Vater using duodenal approach**
          Includes: Operations on ampulla of Vater nec
          *   Papilla of Vater*
          *   Sphincter of Oddi*

J36.1   Excision of ampulla of Vater using duodenal approach
J36.2   Biopsy of lesion of ampulla of Vater using duodenal approach
          Includes: Biopsy of ampulla of Vater using duodenal approach
J36.8   Other specified
J36.9   Unspecified

J37   **Other open operations on bile duct**

J37.1   Open biopsy of lesion of bile duct
         Includes: Open biopsy of bile duct
                  Biopsy of lesion of bile duct
                  Biopsy of bile duct
J37.2   Operative cholangiography through cystic duct
J37.3   Direct puncture operative cholangiography
         Includes: Operative cholangiography nec
J37.4   Operative choledochoscopy nec
J37.8   Other specified
J37.9   Unspecified

J38   **Endoscopic incision of sphincter of Oddi**
         Includes: Endoscopic retrograde incision of sphincter of oddi

J38.1   Endoscopic sphincterotomy of sphincter of Oddi and removal of calculus hfq
J38.2   Endoscopic sphincterotomy of sphincter of Oddi and insertion of tubal prosthesis into bile duct
J38.8   Other specified
J38.9   Unspecified
         Includes: Endoscopic sphincterotomy of papilla of Vater

J39   **Other therapeutic endoscopic operations on ampulla of Vater**
         Includes: Therapeutic endoscopic retrograde operations on ampulla of Vater
                  Papilla of Vater
                  Sphincter of Oddi

J39.1   Endoscopic sphincterotomy of accessory ampulla of Vater
J39.8   Other specified
J39.9   Unspecified

J40   **Endoscopic retrograde placement of prosthesis in bile duct**
         Excludes: When associated with endoscopic sphincterotomy of sphincter of Oddi (J38)

J40.1   Endoscopic retrograde insertion of tubal prosthesis into both hepatic ducts
J40.2   Endoscopic retrograde insertion of tubal prosthesis into bile duct nec
J40.3   Endoscopic retrograde renewal of tubal prosthesis in bile duct
J40.4   Endoscopic retrograde removal of tubal prosthesis from bile duct
J40.8   Other specified
J40.9   Unspecified

J41   **Other therapeutic endoscopic retrograde operations on bile duct**
         Excludes: When associated with endoscopic sphincterotomy of sphincter of Oddi (J38)
         Note: It is not necessary to code additionally any mention of diagnostic endoscopic examination of
                  bile duct (J44.9)

J41.1   Endoscopic retrograde extraction of calculus from bile duct
J41.2   Endoscopic dilation of bile duct nec
         Includes: Endoscopic dilation of stricture of bile duct nec
J41.8   Other specified
J41.9   Unspecified

J42   **Therapeutic endoscopic retrograde operations on pancreatic duct**
         Note: It is not necessary to code additionally any mention of diagnostic endoscopic examination of
                  pancreas (J45.9)

J42.1   Endoscopic retrograde insertion of tubal prosthesis into pancreatic duct
J42.2   Endoscopic retrograde renewal of tubal prosthesis in pancreatic duct
J42.3   Endoscopic retrograde removal of calculus from pancreatic duct
J42.4   Endoscopic retrograde drainage of lesion of pancreas
J42.5   Endoscopic retrograde dilation of pancreatic duct
J42.8   Other specified
J42.9   Unspecified

J43   **Diagnostic endoscopic retrograde examination of bile duct and pancreatic duct**

J43.1   Endoscopic retrograde cholangiopancreatography and biopsy of lesion of ampulla of Vater
         Includes: Endoscopic retrograde cholangiopancreatography and biopsy of ampulla of Vater
J43.2   Endoscopic retrograde cholangiopancreatography and biopsy of lesion of biliary or pancreatic system nec
         Includes: Endoscopic retrograde cholangiopancreatography and biopsy of biliary or pancreatic system
             nec
         Note: *Use subsidiary code for cytology as necessary (Y21)*
                   Use subsidiary site code as necessary
J43.8   Other specified
J43.9   Unspecified
         Includes: Endoscopic retrograde cholangiopancreatography nec

J44   **Diagnostic endoscopic retrograde examination of bile duct**
         Excludes: When associated with diagnostic endoscopic retrograd examination of pancreatic duct (J43)

J44.1   Endoscopic retrograde cholangiography and biopsy of lesion of bile duct
         Includes: Endoscopic retrograde cholangiography and biopsy of bile duct
                 Endoscopic retrograde biopsy of lesion of bile duct
                 Endoscopic retrograde biopsy of bile duct
         Note: *Use subsidiary code for cytology as necessary (Y21)*
J44.8   Other specified
J44.9   Unspecified
         Includes: Endoscopic retrograde cholangiography nec

J45   **Diagnostic endoscopic retrograde examination of pancreatic duct**
         Excludes: When associated with diagnostic endoscopic retrograde examination of bile duct (J43)

J45.1   Endoscopic retrograde pancreatography and biopsy of lesion of pancreas
         Includes: Endoscopic retrograde pancreatography and biopsy of pancreas
                 Endoscopic retrograde biopsy of lesion of pancreas
                 Endoscopic retrograde biopsy of pancreas
         Note: *Use subsidiary code for cytology as necessary (Y21)*
J45.2   Endoscopic retrograde pancreatography and collection of pancreatic juice
         Includes: Endoscopic retrograde collection of pure pancreatic juice
J45.3   Endoscopic retrograde pancreatography through accessory ampulla of vater
J45.8   Other specified
J45.9   Unspecified
         Includes: Endoscopic retrograde pancreatography nec

J46   **Therapeutic percutaneous attention to connection of bile duct**
         Note: *Use subsidiary code to identify method of image control as necessary (Y53)*

J46.1   Percutaneous dilation of anastomosis of bile duct and insertion of tubal prosthesis hfq
J46.2   Percutaneous dilation of anastomosis of bile duct nec
J46.8   Other specified
J46.9   Unspecified

J47   **Therapeutic percutaneous insertion of prosthesis into bile duct**
         Note: *Use subsidiary code to identify method of image control as necessary (Y53)*

J47.1   Percutaneous insertion of tubal prosthesis into both hepatic ducts
J47.2   Percutaneous insertion of tubal prosthesis into right hepatic duct nec
J47.3   Percutaneous insertion of tubal prosthesis into left hepatic duct nec
J47.4   Percutaneous insertion of tubal prosthesis into hepatic duct nec
J47.5   Percutaneous insertion of tubal prosthesis into common bile duct
J47.8   Other specified
J47.9   Unspecified

J48   **Other therapeutic percutaneous operations on bile duct**
            Note: Use subsidiary code to identify method of image control as necessary (Y53)

J48.1   Renewal of percutaneously inserted tubal prosthesis in bile duct
J48.2   Removal of percutaneously inserted tubal prosthesis from bile duct
J48.3   Attention to percutaneously inserted tubal prosthesis in bile duct nec
J48.8   Other specified
J48.9   Unspecified

J49   **Therapeutic operations on bile duct along T tube track**

J49.1   Endoscopic removal of calculus from bile duct along T tube track
        Includes: Removal of calculus from bile duct along T tube track using choledochoscope
J49.2   Percutaneous removal of calculus from bile duct along T tube track
        Includes: Percutaneous removal of calculus from bile duct along T tube track using image control
        Note: Use subsidiary code to identify method of image control as necessary (Y53)
J49.8   Other specified
J49.9   Unspecified

J50   **Percutaneous examination of bile duct**
            Note: Use subsidiary code to identify method of image control as necessary (Y53)

J50.1   T tube cholangiography
J50.2   Percutaneous cholangiography
J50.8   Other specified
J50.9   Unspecified

J52   **Other operations on bile duct**

J52.1   Extracorporeal lithotripsy of calculus in bile duct
J52.8   Other specified
J52.9   Unspecified

J54   **Transplantation of pancreas**

J54.1   Transplantation of pancreas and duodenum
J54.2   Transplantation of whole pancreas
J54.3   Transplantation of tail of pancreas
J54.4   Transplantation of islet of langerhans
J54.5   Renewal of transplanted pancreatic tissue
J54.8   Other specified
J54.9   Unspecified

J55   **Total excision of pancreas**

J55.1   Total pancreatectomy and excision of surrounding tissue
        Note: Use additional code for coincidental transplantation of islet cell tissue (J54.4)
J55.2   Total pancreatectomy nec
J55.3   Excision of transplanted pancreas
J55.8   Other specified
J55.9   Unspecified

J56   **Excision of head of pancreas**

J56.1   Pancreaticoduodenectomy and excision of surrounding tissue
J56.2   Pancreaticoduodenectomy and resection of antrum of stomach
J56.3   Pancreaticoduodenectomy nec
J56.8   Other specified
J56.9   Unspecified

J57 Other partial excision of pancreas

J57.1 Subtotal pancreatectomy
J57.2 Left pancreatectomy and drainage of pancreatic duct
J57.3 Left pancreatectomy nec
J57.4 Excision of tail of pancreas and drainage of pancreatic duct
J57.5 Excision of tail of pancreas nec
J57.8 Other specified
J57.9 Unspecified
Includes: Pancreatectomy nec

J58 Extirpation of lesion of pancreas

J58.1 Excision of lesion of islet of langerhans
J58.2 Excision of lesion of pancreas nec
J58.3 Destruction of lesion of pancreas
J58.8 Other specified
J58.9 Unspecified

J59 Connection of pancreatic duct

J59.1 Anastomosis of pancreatic duct to stomach
J59.2 Anastomosis of pancreatic duct to duodenum
J59.3 Anastomosis of pancreatic duct to transposed jejunum
J59.4 Anastomosis of pancreatic duct to jejunum nec
J59.5 Revision of anastomosis of pancreatic duct
J59.6 Closure of anastomosis of pancreatic duct
J59.8 Other specified
J59.9 Unspecified

J60 Other open operations on pancreatic duct

J60.1 Drainage of pancreatic duct
J60.2 Open removal of calculus from pancreatic duct
Includes: Removal of calculus from pancreatic duct nec
J60.3 Insertion of T tube into pancreatic duct
J60.4 Open insertion of tubal prosthesis into pancreatic duct
Includes: Insertion of tubal prosthesis into pancreatic duct nec
J60.5 Open dilation of pancreatic duct
Includes: Dilation of pancreatic duct nec
J60.8 Other specified
J60.9 Unspecified

J61 Open drainage of lesion of pancreas

J61.1 Open cystogastrotomy of pancreas
J61.2 Drainage of cyst of pancreas into transposed jejunum
J61.3 Drainage of cyst of pancreas into jejunum nec
J61.4 Drainage of cyst of pancreas nec
J61.8 Other specified
J61.9 Unspecified

J62 Incision of pancreas

J62.1 Division of annular pancreas
J62.8 Other specified
J62.9 Unspecified

J63 Open examination of pancreas

J63.1 Open pancreatography through tail of pancreas
J63.2 Open pancreatography through papilla of Vater
J63.3 Open pancreatography nec
J63.8 Other specified
J63.9 Unspecified

J65	**Other open operations on pancreas**

J65.1	Open biopsy of lesion of pancreas
	Includes: Open biopsy of pancreas
	Biopsy of lesion of pancreas nec
	Biopsy of pancreas nec
J65.8	Other specified
J65.9	Unspecified

J66	**Therapeutic percutaneous operations on pancreas**
	Note: Use subsidiary code to identify method of image control as necessary (Y53)

J66.1	Percutaneous drainage of lesion of pancreas and insertion of cystogastrostomy tube nec
J66.2	Percutaneous drainage of lesion of pancreas and insertion of temporary external drain hfq
J66.3	Percutaneous drainage of lesion of pancreas nec
J66.4	Percutaneous aspiration of lesion of pancreas
J66.8	Other specified
J66.9	Unspecified

J67	**Diagnostic percutaneous operations on pancreas**
	Note: Use subsidiary code to identify method of image control as necessary (Y53)

J67.1	Diagnostic percutaneous aspiration of lesion of pancreas
J67.2	Percutaneous puncture of pancreatic duct and pancreatography
J67.8	Other specified
J67.9	Unspecified

J69	**Total excision of spleen**

J69.1	Total excision of spleen and replantation of fragments of spleen
J69.2	Total splenectomy
J69.3	Excision of accessory spleen
J69.8	Other specified
J69.9	Unspecified
	Includes: Splenectomy nec

J70	**Other excision of spleen**

J70.1	Partial splenectomy
J70.2	Marsupialisation of lesion of spleen
J70.8	Other specified
J70.9	Unspecified

J72	**Other operations on spleen**

J72.1	Transplantation of spleen
J72.2	Embolisation of spleen
J72.3	Biopsy of lesion of spleen
	Includes: Biopsy of spleen
J72.4	Repair of spleen
J72.5	Banding of spleen
J72.8	Other specified
J72.9	Unspecified

K01   **Transplantation of heart and lung**

K01.1   Allotransplantation of heart and lung
K01.2   Revision of transplantation of heart and lung
K01.8   Other specified
K01.9   Unspecified

K02   **Other transplantation of heart**

K02.1   Allotransplantation of heart nec
K02.2   Xenotransplantation of heart
K02.3   Implantation of prosthetic heart
K02.4   Piggy back transplantation of heart
K02.5   Revision of implantation of prosthetic heart
K02.6   Revision of transplantation of heart nec
K02.8   Other specified
K02.9   Unspecified

K04   **Correction of tetralogy of fallot**
      Note: *Do not use secondary code for concurrent closure of defect of septum of heart or construction of cardiac conduit*

K04.1   Correction of tetralogy of fallot using valved right ventricular outflow conduit
K04.2   Correction of tetralogy of fallot using right ventricular outflow conduit nec
K04.3   Correction of tetralogy of fallot using right ventricular outflow patch
K04.4   Revision of correction of tetralogy of fallot
K04.8   Other specified
K04.9   Unspecified

K05   **Atrial inversion operations for transposition of great vessels**
      Note: *Use supplementary code for concurrent correction of other associated abnormality*

K05.1   Reconstruction of atrium using atrial patch for transposition of great vessels
K05.2   Reconstruction of atrium using atrial wall for transposition of great vessels
K05.8   Other specified
K05.9   Unspecified

K06   **Other correction of transposition of great vessels**
      Note: *Use supplementary code for concurrent correction of other associated abnormality*

K06.1   Repositioning of transposed great vessels
K06.8   Other specified
K06.9   Unspecified

K07   **Correction of total anomalous pulmonary venous connection**

K07.1   Correction of total anomalous pulmonary venous connection to supracardiac vessel
K07.2   Correction of total anomalous pulmonary venous connection to coronary sinus
K07.3   Correction of total anomalous pulmonary venous connection to infradiaphragmatic vessel
K07.8   Other specified
K07.9   Unspecified

K09 **Closure of defect of atrioventricular septum**
Excludes: When associated with correction of tetralogy of fallot (K04)

K09.1   Closure of defect of atrioventricular septum using dual prosthetic patches
K09.2   Closure of defect of atrioventricular septum using prosthetic patch nec
K09.3   Closure of defect of atrioventricular septum using tissue graft
K09.4   Closure of persistent ostium primum
K09.5   Primary closure of defect of atrioventricular septum nec
K09.6   Revision of closure of defect of atrioventricular septum
K09.8   Other specified
K09.9   Unspecified

K10 **Closure of defect of interatrial septum**
Excludes: When associated with correction of tetralogy of fallot (K04)

K10.1   Closure of defect of interatrial septum using prosthetic patch
K10.2   Closure of defect of interatrial septum using pericardial patch
K10.3   Closure of defect of interatrial septum using tissue graft nec
K10.4   Primary closure of defect of interatrial septum nec
K10.5   Revision of closure of defect of interatrial septum
K10.8   Other specified
K10.9   Unspecified

K11 **Closure of defect of interventricular septum**
Excludes: When associated with correction of tetralogy of Fallot (K04)

K11.1   Closure of defect of interventricular septum using prosthetic patch
K11.2   Closure of defect of interventricular septum using pericardial patch
K11.3   Closure of defect of interventricular septum using tissue graft nec
K11.4   Primary closure of defect of interventricular septum nec
K11.5   Revision of closure of defect of interventricular septum
K11.8   Other specified
K11.9   Unspecified

K12 **Closure of defect of unspecified septum of heart**
Excludes: When associated with correction of tetralogy of Fallot (K04)

K12.1   Closure of defect of septum of heart using prosthetic patch nec
K12.2   Closure of defect of septum of heart using pericardial patch nec
K12.3   Closure of defect of septum of heart using tissue graft nec
K12.4   Primary closure of defect of septum of heart nec
K12.5   Revision of closure of septum of heart nec
K12.8   Other specified
K12.9   Unspecified

K14 **Other open operations on septum of heart**

K14.1   Open enlargement of defect of atrial septum
K14.2   Open atrial septostomy
         Includes: Atrial septostomy nec
K14.8   Other specified
K14.9   Unspecified

K15 **Closed operations on septum of heart**

K15.1   Closed enlargement of defect of atrial septum
K15.2   Closed atrial septostomy
K15.8   Other specified
K15.9   Unspecified

K16 **Therapeutic transluminal operations on septum of heart**

K16.1   Percutaneous transluminal balloon atrial septostomy
K16.2   Percutaneous transluminal atrial septostomy nec
K16.8   Other specified
K16.9   Unspecified

K18   **Creation of valved cardiac conduit**
Excludes: When associated with correction of tetralogy of Fallot (K04)

K18.1   Creation of valved conduit between atrium and ventricle of heart
K18.2   Creation of valved conduit between right atrium and pulmonary artery
K18.3   Creation of valved conduit between right ventricle of heart and pulmonary artery
K18.4   Creation of valved conduit between left ventricle of heart and aorta
K18.5   Revision of valved cardiac conduit
K18.8   Other specified
K18.9   Unspecified

K19   **Creation of other cardiac conduit**
Excludes: When associated with correction of tetralogy of Fallot (K04)

K19.1   Creation of conduit between atrium and ventricle of heart nec
K19.2   Creation of conduit between right atrium and pulmonary artery nec
K19.3   Creation of conduit between right ventricle of heart and pulmonary artery nec
K19.4   Creation of conduit between right ventricle of heart and vena cava
K19.5   Creation of conduit between left ventricle of heart and aorta nec
K19.6   Revision of cardiac conduit nec
K19.8   Other specified
K19.9   Unspecified

K20   **Refashioning of atrium**

K20.1   Correction of persistent sinus venosus
K20.2   Correction of partial anomalous pulmonary venous drainage
K20.8   Other specified
K20.9   Unspecified

K22   **Other operations on wall of atrium**
Excludes: Operations on coronary artery (K40-K51) or conducting system of heart (K52 K57-K58)

K22.1   Excision of lesion of atrium
K22.2   Repair of atrium nec
K22.8   Other specified
K22.9   Unspecified

K23   **Other operations of wall of heart**
Excludes: Operations on coronary artery (K40-K51) or conducting system of heart (K52 K57-K58)

K23.1   Excision of lesion of wall of heart nec
        Includes: Excision of lesion of ventricle of heart
K23.2   Biopsy of lesion of wall of heart
        Includes: Biopsy of wall of heart
                 Biopsy of lesion of heart nec
                 Biopsy of heart nec
K23.3   Repair of wall of heart nec
K23.4   Revascularisation of wall of heart
        Includes: Revascularisation of heart
K23.8   Other specified
K23.9   Unspecified

K25   **Plastic repair of mitral valve**
Note: Use supplementary code for concurrent multiple replacement of valves of heart (eg K26)
*   Use as supplementary code when associated with bypass of coronary artery (K40-K46)*

K25.1   Allograft replacement of mitral valve
K25.2   Xenograft replacement of mitral valve
K25.3   Prosthetic replacement of mitral valve
K25.4   Replacement of mitral valve nec
K25.5   Mitral valvuloplasty nec
K25.8   Other specified
K25.9   Unspecified

K26   Plastic repair of aortic valve
Note: Use supplementary code for concurrent multiple replacement of valves of heart (eg K25)
Use as supplementary code when associated with bypass of coronary artery (K40-K46)

K26.1   Allograft replacement of aortic valve
K26.2   Xenograft replacement of aortic valve
K26.3   Prosthetic replacement of aortic valve
K26.4   Replacement of aortic valve nec
K26.5   Aortic valvuloplasty nec
K26.8   Other specified
K26.9   Unspecified

K27   Plastic repair of tricuspid valve
Note: Use supplementary code for concurrent multiple replacement of valves of heart (eg K28)
Use as supplementary code when associated with bypass of coronary artery (K40-K46)

K27.1   Allograft replacement of tricuspid valve
K27.2   Xenograft replacement of tricuspid valve
K27.3   Prosthetic replacement of tricuspid valve
K27.4   Replacement of tricuspid valve nec
K27.5   Repositioning of tricuspid valve
K27.6   Tricuspid valvuloplasty nec
K27.8   Other specified
K27.9   Unspecified

K28   Plastic repair of pulmonary valve
Note: Use supplementary code for concurrent multiple replacement of valves of heart (eg K27)
Use as supplementary code when associated with bypass of coronary artery (K40-K46)

K28.1   Allograft replacement of pulmonary valve
K28.2   Xenograft replacement of pulmonary valve
K28.3   Prosthetic replacement of pulmonary valve
K28.4   Replacement of pulmonary valve nec
K28.5   Pulmonary valvuloplasty nec
K28.8   Other specified
K28.9   Unspecified

K29   Plastic repair of unspecified valve of heart
Note: Use as supplementary code when associated with bypass of coronary artery (K40-K46)

K29.1   Allograft replacement of valve of heart nec
K29.2   Xenograft replacement of valve of heart nec
K29.3   Prosthetic replacement of valve of heart nec
K29.4   Replacement of valve of heart nec
K29.5   Valvuloplasty of heart nec
K29.8   Other specified
K29.9   Unspecified

K30   Revision of plastic repair of valve of heart
Includes: Revision of replacement of valve of heart

K30.1   Revision of plastic repair of mitral valve
K30.2   Revision of plastic repair of aortic valve
K30.3   Revision of plastic repair of tricuspid valve
K30.4   Revision of plastic repair of pulmonary valve
K30.8   Other specified
K30.9   Unspecified

K31 **Open incision of valve of heart**
Includes: Incision of valve of heart nec

K31.1   Open mitral valvotomy
K31.2   Open aortic valvotomy
K31.3   Open tricuspid valvotomy
K31.4   Open pulmonary valvotomy
K31.8   Other specified
K31.9   Unspecified
Includes: Valvotomy nec

K32 **Closed incision of valve of heart**

K32.1   Closed mitral valvotomy
K32.2   Closed aortic valvotomy
K32.3   Closed tricuspid valvotomy
K32.4   Closed pulmonary valvotomy
K32.8   Other specified
K32.9   Unspecified

K34 **Other open operations on valve of heart**

K34.1   Annuloplasty of mitral valve
K34.2   Annuloplasty of tricuspid valve
K34.3   Annuloplasty of valve of heart nec
K34.4   Excision of vegetations of valve of heart
K34.8   Other specified
K34.9   Unspecified

K35 **Therapeutic transluminal operations on valve of heart**

K35.1   Percutaneous transluminal mitral valvotomy
K35.2   Percutaneous transluminal aortic valvotomy
K35.3   Percutaneous transluminal tricuspid valvotomy
K35.4   Percutaneous transluminal pulmonary valvotomy
K35.5   Percutaneous transluminal valvuloplasty
K35.8   Other specified
K35.9   Unspecified

K37 **Removal of obstruction from structure adjacent to valve of heart**
Excludes: Cardiac conduit operations (K18 K19)

K37.1   Infundibulectomy of heart using patch
K37.2   Infundibulectomy of heart nec
K37.3   Repair of subaortic stenosis
K37.4   Repair of supraaortic stenosis
K37.8   Other specified
K37.9   Unspecified

K38 **Other operations on structure adjacent to valve of heart**

K38.1   Operations on papillary muscle
K38.2   Operations on chordae tendineae
K38.8   Other specified
K38.9   Unspecified

K40   **Saphenous vein graft replacement of coronary artery**
Note: *Use supplementary code for concurrent repair or replacement of valve of heart (K25-K29)*
            Use supplementary code for concurrent excision of lesion of ventricle of heart (K23.1) or
            closure of defect of interventricular septum (K11)

K40.1   Saphenous vein graft replacement of one coronary artery
K40.2   Saphenous vein graft replacement of two coronary arteries
K40.3   Saphenous vein graft replacement of three coronary arteries
K40.4   Saphenous vein graft replacement of four or more coronary arteries
K40.8   Other specified
K40.9   Unspecified

K41   **Other autograft replacement of coronary artery**
Note: *Use supplementary code for concurrent repair or replacement of valve of heart (K25-K29)*
            Use supplementary code for concurrent excision of lesion of ventricle of heart (K23.1) or
            closure of defect of interventricular septum (K11)

K41.1   Autograft replacement of one coronary artery nec
K41.2   Autograft replacement of two coronary arteries nec
K41.3   Autograft replacement of three coronary arteries nec
K41.4   Autograft replacement of four or more coronary arteries nec
K41.8   Other specified
K41.9   Unspecified

K42   **Allograft replacement of coronary artery**
Note: *Use supplementary code for concurrent repair or replacement of valve of heart (K25-K29)*
            Use supplementary code for concurrent excision of lesion of ventricle of heart (K23.1) or
            closure of defect of interventricular septum (K11)

K42.1   Allograft replacement of one coronary artery
K42.2   Allograft replacement of two coronary arteries
K42.3   Allograft replacement of three coronary arteries
K42.4   Allograft replacement of four or more coronary arteries
K42.8   Other specified
K42.9   Unspecified

K43   **Prosthetic replacement of coronary artery**
Note: *Use supplementary code for concurrent repair or replacement of valve of heart (K25-K29)*
            Use supplementary code for concurrent excision of lesion of ventricle of heart (K23.1) or
            closure of defect of interventricular septum (K11)

K43.1   Prosthetic replacement of one coronary artery
K43.2   Prosthetic replacement of two coronary arteries
K43.3   Prosthetic replacement of three coronary arteries
K43.4   Prosthetic replacement of four or more coronary arteries
K43.8   Other specified
K43.9   Unspecified

K44   **Other replacement of coronary artery**
Includes: Coronary artery bypass graft nec
Note: *Use supplementary code for concurrent repair or replacement of valve of heart (K25-K29)*
            Use supplementary code for concurrent excision of lesion of ventricle of heart (K23.1) or
            closure of defect of interventricular septum (K11)

K44.1   Replacement of coronary arteries using multiple methods
K44.2   Revision of replacement of coronary artery
K44.8   Other specified
K44.9   Unspecified

K45   **Connection of thoracic artery to coronary artery**

K45.1   Double anastomosis of mammary arteries to coronary arteries
K45.2   Double anastomosis of thoracic arteries to coronary arteries nec
K45.3   Anastomosis of mammary artery to left anterior descending coronary artery
K45.4   Anastomosis of mammary artery to coronary artery nec
K45.5   Anastomosis of thoracic artery to coronary artery nec
K45.6   Revision of connection of thoracic artery to coronary artery
K45.8   Other specified
K45.9   Unspecified

K46   **Other bypass of coronary artery**
Excludes: Coronary artery bypass graft (K40-K44)

K46.1   Double implantation of mammary arteries into heart
K46.2   Double implantation of thoracic arteries into heart nec
K46.3   Implantation of mammary artery into heart nec
K46.4   Implantation of thoracic artery into heart nec
K46.5   Revision of implantation of thoracic artery into heart
K46.8   Other specified
K46.9   Unspecified

K47   **Repair of coronary artery**

K47.1   Endarterectomy of coronary artery
K47.2   Repair of arteriovenous fistula of coronary artery
K47.3   Repair of aneurysm of coronary artery
K47.8   Other specified
K47.9   Unspecified

K48   **Other open operations on coronary artery**

K48.1   Transection of muscle bridge of coronary artery
K48.2   Transposition of coronary artery nec
K48.3   Open angioplasty of coronary artery
K48.4   Exploration of coronary artery
K48.8   Other specified
K48.9   Unspecified

K49   **Transluminal balloon angioplasty of coronary artery**

K49.1   Percutaneous transluminal balloon angioplasty of one coronary artery
Includes: Angioplasty of coronary artery nec
K49.2   Percutaneous transluminal balloon angioplasty of multiple coronary arteries
K49.3   Percutaneous transluminal balloon angioplasty of bypass graft of coronary artery
K49.8   Other specified
K49.9   Unspecified

K50   **Other therapeutic transluminal operations on coronary artery**

K50.1   Percutaneous transluminal laser coronary angioplasty
K50.2   Percutaneous transluminal coronary thrombolysis using streptokinase
K50.3   Percutaneous transluminal injection of therapeutic substance into coronary artery nec
K50.8   Other specified
K50.9   Unspecified

K51   **Diagnostic transluminal operations on coronary artery**

K51.1   Percutaneous transluminal angioscopy
K51.8   Other specified
K51.9   Unspecified

K52 Open operations on conducting system of heart

K52.1 Open ablation of atrioventricular node
      Includes: Ablation of atrioventricular node nec
K52.2 Epicardial excision of rhythmogenic focus
K52.3 Endocardial excision of rhythmogenic focus
K52.4 Open division of accessory pathway within heart
K52.5 Open division of conducting system of heart nec
K52.8 Other specified
K52.9 Unspecified

K53 Other incision of heart

K53.1 Inspection of valve of heart
K53.2 Exploration of heart nec
K53.8 Other specified
K53.9 Unspecified
      Includes: Cardiotomy nec

K55 Other open operations on heart

K55.1 Ligation of sinus of valsalva
K55.2 Open chest massage of heart
K55.8 Other specified
K55.9 Unspecified

K56 Transluminal heart assist operations

K56.1 Transluminal insertion of pulsation balloon into aorta
K56.2 Transluminal insertion of heart assist system nec
K56.3 Transluminal maintenance of heart assist system
K56.4 Transluminal removal of heart assist system
K56.8 Other specified
K56.9 Unspecified

K57 Other therapeutic transluminal operations on heart

K57.1 Percutaneous transluminal ablation of atrioventricular node
K57.2 Percutaneous transluminal ablation of conducting system of heart nec
K57.8 Other specified
K57.9 Unspecified

K58 Diagnostic transluminal operations on heart

K58.1 Percutaneous transluminal mapping of conducting system of heart
K58.2 Percutaneous transluminal electrophysiological studies on conducting system of heart
K58.8 Other specified
K58.9 Unspecified

K60 Cardiac pacemaker system introduced through vein
      Includes: Automatic cardioverter introduced through vein
              Automatic cardiac defibrillator introduced through vein

K60.1 Implantation of intravenous cardiac pacemaker system
K60.2 Resiting of lead of intravenous cardiac pacemaker system
K60.3 Renewal of intravenous cardiac pacemaker system
      Includes: Renewal of battery of intravenous cardiac pacemaker system
              Maintenance of intravenous cardiac pacemaker system nec
K60.4 Removal of intravenous cardiac pacemaker system
K60.8 Other specified
K60.9 Unspecified

K61 Other cardiac pacemaker system
Includes: Automatic cardioverter
Automatic cardiac defibrillator

K61.1 Implantation of cardiac pacemaker system nec
K61.2 Resiting of lead of cardiac pacemaker system nec
K61.3 Renewal of cardiac pacemaker system nec
Includes: Renewal of battery of cardiac pacemaker system nec
Maintenance of cardiac pacemaker system nec
K61.4 Removal of cardiac pacemaker system nec
K61.8 Other specified
K61.9 Unspecified

K63 Contrast radiology of heart

K63.1 Angiocardiography of combination of right and left side of heart
K63.2 Angiocardiography of right side of heart nec
K63.3 Angiocardiography of left side of heart nec
K63.4 Coronary arteriography using two catheters
K63.5 Coronary arteriography using single catheter
K63.6 Coronary arteriography nec
K63.8 Other specified
K63.9 Unspecified

K65 Catheterisation of heart

K65.1 Catheterisation of combination of right and left side of heart nec
K65.2 Catheterisation of right side of heart nec
K65.3 Catheterisation of left side of heart nec
K65.8 Other specified
K65.9 Unspecified

K66 Other operations on heart

K66.1 Cardiotachygraphy
K66.8 Other specified
K66.9 Unspecified

K67 Excision of pericardium

K67.1 Excision of lesion of pericardium
K67.8 Other specified
K67.9 Unspecified

K68 Drainage of pericardium

K68.1 Decompression of cardiac tamponade
K68.2 Pericardiocentesis nec
K68.8 Other specified
K68.9 Unspecified

K69 Incision of pericardium

K69.1 Freeing of adhesions of pericardium
K69.2 Fenestration of pericardium
K69.8 Other specified
K69.9 Unspecified

K71 Other operations on pericardium

K71.1 Biopsy of lesion of pericardium
Includes: Biopsy of pericardium
K71.2 Repair of pericardium
K71.3 Injection of therapeutic substance into pericardium
K71.4 Exploration of pericardium
K71.8 Other specified
K71.9 Unspecified

CHAPTER L

ARTERIES AND VEINS

(CODES L01-L97)

Note: *This chapter contains certain specified arteries and veins*

This specification does not extend beyond the actual named vessel

Smaller branches or tributaries of the above are to be coded to the other and unspecified vessel categories with an appropriate site code where available

L01   Open operations for combined abnormality of great vessels

L01.1   Correction of persistent truncus arteriosus
        Note: Do not code closure of defect of septum of heart separately
L01.2   Application of band to persistent truncus arteriosus
L01.3   Repair of hemitruncus arteriosus
L01.4   Closure of aortopulmonary window
L01.8   Other specified
L01.9   Unspecified

L02   Open correction of patent ductus arteriosus

L02.1   Division of patent ductus ateriosus
L02.2   Ligature of patent ductus arteriosus
L02.3   Closure of patent ductus arteriosus nec
L02.4   Revision of correction of patent ductus arteriosus
L02.8   Other specified
L02.9   Unspecified

L03   Transluminal operations on abnormality of great vessel

L03.1   Percutaneous transluminal prosthetic occlusion of patent ductus arteriosus
L03.8   Other specified
L03.9   Unspecified

L05   Creation of shunt to pulmonary artery from aorta using interposition tube prosthesis

L05.1   Creation of shunt to main pulmonary artery from ascending aorta using interposition tube prosthesis
L05.2   Creation of shunt to right pulmonary artery from ascending aorta using interposition tube prosthesis
L05.3   Creation of shunt to left pulmonary artery from ascending aorta using interposition tube prosthesis
L05.8   Other specified
L05.9   Unspecified

L06   Other connection to pulmonary artery from aorta

L06.1   Creation of aortopulmonary window
L06.2   Creation of anastomosis to main pulmonary artery from ascending aorta nec
L06.3   Creation of anastomosis to right pulmonary artery from ascending aorta nec
L06.4   Creation of anastomosis to left pulmonary artery from descending aorta nec
L06.5   Creation of anastomosis to pulmonary artery from aorta nec
L06.6   Revision of anastomosis to pulmonary artery from aorta
L06.8   Other specified
L06.9   Unspecified

L07 **Creation of shunt to pulmonary artery from subclavian artery using interposition tube prosthesis**

L07.1 Creation of shunt to right pulmonary artery from right subclavian artery using interposition tube prosthesis
L07.2 Creation of shunt to left pulmonary artery from left subclavian artery using interposition tube prosthesis
L07.8 Other specified
L07.9 Unspecified

L08 **Other connection to pulmonary artery from subclavian artery**

L08.1 Creation of anastomosis to right pulmonary artery from right subclavian artery nec
L08.2 Creation of anastomosis to left pulmonary artery from left subclavian artery nec
L08.3 Creation of anastomosis to pulmonary artery from subclavian artery nec
L08.4 Revision of anastomosis to pulmonary artery from subclavian artery
L08.8 Other specified
L08.9 Unspecified

L09 **Other connection to pulmonary artery**

L09.1 Creation of anastomosis to pulmonary artery from vena cava
L09.2 Removal of anastomosis between pulmonary artery and vena cava
L09.8 Other specified
L09.9 Unspecified

L10 **Repair of pulmonary artery**
   Note: Use supplementary code for concurrent operations on pulmonary valve (K28 K30-K35)

L10.1 Repair of pulmonary artery using prosthesis
L10.2 Repair of pulmonary artery using patch
L10.3 Repair of anomalous pulmonary artery nec
L10.8 Other specified
L10.9 Unspecified

L12 **Other open operations on pulmonary artery**

L12.1 Application of band to pulmonary artery
L12.2 Adjustment of band to pulmonary artery
L12.3 Removal of band from pulmonary artery
L12.4 Open embolectomy of pulmonary artery
   Includes: Open thrombectomy of pulmonary artery
   Embolectomy of pulmonary artery nec
   Thrombectomy of pulmonary artery nec
L12.5 Open embolisation of pulmonary artery
L12.8 Other specified
L12.9 Unspecified

L13 **Transluminal operations on pulmonary artery**

L13.1 Percutaneous transluminal embolectomy of pulmonary artery
   Includes: Percutaneous transluminal thrombectomy of pulmonary artery
L13.2 Percutaneous transluminal embolisation of pulmonary artery
   Includes: Embolisation of pulmonary artery nec
L13.3 Arteriography of pulmonary artery
L13.8 Other specified
L13.9 Unspecified

L16 **Extraanatomic bypass of aorta**
Note: In categories L16-L21 reference to iliac artery (nfq) should be understood to include:
Common iliac artery
External iliac artery
Internal iliac artery
Similarly reference to femoral artery includes:
Common femoral artery
Deep femoral artery
Superficial femoral artery

L16.1   Emergency bypass of aorta by anastomosis of axillary artery to femoral artery
L16.2   Bypass of aorta by anastomosis of axillary artery to femoral artery nec
L16.8   Other specified
L16.9   Unspecified

L18 **Emergency replacement of aneurysmal segment of aorta**
Note at L16 applies
Includes: Emergency replacement of aneurysmal segment of aorta using prosthesis

L18.1   Emergency replacement of aneurysmal segment of ascending aorta by anastomosis of aorta to aorta
Note: Use supplementary code for concurrent operations on aortic valve (K26 K30-K35)
L18.2   Emergency replacement of aneurysmal segment of thoracic aorta by anastomosis of aorta to aorta nec
L18.3   Emergency replacement of aneurysmal segment of suprarenal abdominal aorta by anastomosis of aorta to aorta
L18.4   Emergency replacement of aneurysmal segment of infrarenal abdominal aorta by anastomosis of aorta to aorta
L18.5   Emergency replacement of aneurysmal segment of abdominal aorta by anastomosis of aorta to aorta nec
L18.6   Emergency replacement of aneurysmal bifurcation of aorta by anastomosis of aorta to iliac artery
L18.8   Other specified
L18.9   Unspecified

L19 **Other replacement of aneurysmal segment of aorta**
Note at L16 applies
Includes: Replacement of aneurysmal segment of aorta using prosthesis nec

L19.1   Replacement of aneurysmal segment of ascending aorta by anastomosis of aorta to aorta nec
Note: Use supplementary code for concurrent operations on aortic valve (K26 K30-K35)
L19.2   Replacement of aneurysmal segment of thoracic aorta by anastomosis of aorta to aorta nec
L19.3   Replacement of aneurysmal segment of suprarenal abdominal aorta by anastomosis of aorta to aorta nec
L19.4   Replacement of aneurysmal segment of infrarenal abdominal aorta by anastomosis of aorta to aorta nec
L19.5   Replacement of aneurysmal segment of abdominal aorta by anastomosis of aorta to aorta nec
L19.6   Replacement of aneurysmal bifurcation of aorta by anastomosis of aorta to iliac artery nec
L19.8   Other specified
L19.9   Unspecified

L20 **Other emergency bypass of segment of aorta**
Note at L16 applies
Includes: Emergency bypass of segment of aorta using prosthesis nec
Emergency replacement of segment of aorta nec
Emergency replacement of segment of aorta using prosthesis nec

L20.1   Emergency bypass of segment of ascending aorta by anastomosis of aorta to aorta nec
Note: Use supplementary code for concurrent operations on aortic valve (K26 K30-K35)
L20.2   Emergency bypass of segment of thoracic aorta by anastomosis of aorta to aorta nec
L20.3   Emergency bypass of segment of suprarenal abdominal aorta by anastomosis of aorta to aorta nec
L20.4   Emergency bypass of segment of infrarenal abdominal aorta by anastomosis of aorta to aorta nec
L20.5   Emergency bypass of segment of abdominal aorta by anastomosis of aorta to aorta nec
L20.6   Emergency bypass of bifurcation of aorta by anastomosis of aorta to iliac artery nec
L20.8   Other specified
L20.9   Unspecified

L21   **Other bypass of segment of aorta**
Note at L16 applies
Includes: Bypass of segment of aorta using prosthesis nec
Replacement of segment of aorta nec
Replacement of segment of aorta using prosthesis nec

L21.1   Bypass of segment of ascending aorta by anastomosis of aorta to aorta nec
Note: Use supplementary code for concurrent operations on aortic valve (K26 K30-K35)
L21.2   Bypass of segment of thoracic aorta by anastomosis of aorta to aorta nec
L21.3   Bypass of segment of suprarenal abdominal aorta by anastomosis of aorta to aorta nec
L21.4   Bypass of segment of infrarenal abdominal aorta by anastomosis of aorta to aorta nec
L21.5   Bypass of segment of abdominal aorta by anastomosis of aorta to aorta nec
L21.6   Bypass of bifurcation of aorta by anastomosis of aorta to iliac artery nec
L21.8   Other specified
L21.9   Unspecified

L22   **Attention to prosthesis of aorta**

L22.1   Revision of prosthesis of thoracic aorta
L22.2   Revision of prosthesis of bifurcation of aorta
L22.3   Revision of prosthesis of abdominal aorta nec
L22.4   Removal of prosthesis from aorta
L22.8   Other specified
L22.9   Unspecified

L23   **Plastic repair of aorta**

L23.1   Plastic repair of aorta and end to end anastomosis of aorta
L23.2   Plastic repair of aorta using subclavian flap
L23.3   Plastic repair of aorta using patch graft
L23.4   Release of vascular ring of aorta
L23.5   Revision of plastic repair of aorta
L23.8   Other specified
L23.9   Unspecified

L25   **Other open operations on aorta**
Includes: Aortic body (L25.5)

L25.1   Endarterectomy of aorta and patch repair of aorta
L25.2   Endarterectomy of aorta nec
L25.3   Open embolectomy of bifurcation of aorta
Includes: Open thrombectomy of bifurcation of aorta
Embolectomy of bifurcation of aorta nec
Thrombectomy of bifurcation of aorta nec
L25.4   Operations on aneurysm of aorta nec
L25.5   Operations on aortic body
L25.8   Other specified
L25.9   Unspecified

L26   **Transluminal operations on aorta**

L26.1   Percutaneous transluminal balloon angioplasty of aorta
L26.2   Percutaneous transluminal angioplasty of aorta nec
L26.3   Percutaneous transluminal embolectomy of bifurcation of aorta
Includes: Percutaneous transluminal thrombectomy of bifurcation of aorta
L26.4   Aortography
L26.8   Other specified
L26.9   Unspecified

L29   **Reconstruction of carotid artery**

L29.1   Replacement of carotid artery using graft
L29.2   Intracranial bypass to carotid artery
L29.3   Bypass to carotid artery nec
L29.4   Endarterectomy of carotid artery and patch repair of carotid artery
L29.5   Endarterectomy of carotid artery nec
L29.8   Other specified
L29.9   Unspecified

L30   **Other open operations on carotid artery**
Includes: Carotid body (L30.5)

L30.1   Repair of carotid artery nec
L30.2   Ligation of carotid artery
L30.3   Open embolectomy of carotid artery
        Includes: Open thrombectomy of carotid artery
                   Embolectomy of carotid artery nec
                   Thrombectomy of carotid artery nec
L30.4   Operations on aneurysm of carotid artery
L30.5   Operations on carotid body
L30.8   Other specified
L30.9   Unspecified

L31   **Transluminal operations on carotid artery**

L31.1   Percutaneous transluminal angioplasty of carotid artery
L31.2   Arteriography of carotid artery
L31.8   Other specified
L31.9   Unspecified

L33   **Operations on aneurysm of cerebral artery**
Includes: Artery of circle of Willis

L33.1   Excision of aneurysm of cerebral artery
L33.2   Clipping of aneurysm of cerebral artery
L33.3   Ligation of aneurysm of cerebral artery nec
L33.4   Obliteration of aneurysm of cerebral artery nec
L33.8   Other specified
L33.9   Unspecified

L34   **Other open operations on cerebral artery**
Includes: Artery of circle of Willis

L34.1   Reconstruction of cerebral artery
L34.2   Anastomosis of cerebral artery
L34.3   Open embolectomy of cerebral artery
        Includes: Open thrombectomy of cerebral artery
                   Embolectomy of cerebral artery nec
                   Thrombectomy of cerebral artery nec
L34.4   Open embolisation of cerebral artery
L34.8   Other specified
L34.9   Unspecified

L35   **Transluminal operations on cerebral artery**
Includes: Artery of circle of Willis

L35.1   Percutaneous transluminal embolisation of cerebral artery
        Includes: Embolisation of cerebral artery nec
L35.2   Arteriography of cerebral artery
L35.8   Other specified
L35.9   Unspecified

L37   **Reconstruction of subclavian artery**
Includes: Axillary artery
             Brachial artery
             Vertebral artery

L37.1   Bypass of subclavian artery nec
L37.2   Endarterectomy of vertebral artery
L37.3   Endarterectomy of subclavian artery and patch repair of subclavian artery
L37.4   Endarterectomy of subclavian artery nec
L37.8   Other specified
L37.9   Unspecified

L38   **Other open operations on subclavian artery**
Includes: Axillary artery
Brachial artery
Vertebral artery

L38.1   Repair of subclavian artery nec
L38.2   Ligation of subclavian artery
L38.3   Open embolectomy of subclavian artery
Includes: Open thrombectomy of subclavian artery
Embolectomy of subclavian artery nec
Thrombectomy of subclavian artery nec
L38.4   Operations on aneurysm of subclavian artery
L38.8   Other specified
L38.9   Unspecified

L39   **Transluminal operations on subclavian artery**
Includes: Axillary artery
Brachial artery
Vertebral artery

L39.1   Percutaneous transluminal angioplasty of subclavian artery
L39.2   Percutaneous transluminal embolectomy of subclavian artery
Includes: Percutaneous transluminal thrombectomy of subclavian artery
L39.3   Percutaneous transluminal embolisation of subclavian artery
Includes: Embolisation of subclavian artery nec
L39.4   Arteriography of subclavian artery
L39.8   Other specified
L39.9   Unspecified

L41   **Reconstruction of renal artery**

L41.1   Plastic repair of renal artery and end to end anastomosis of renal artery
L41.2   Bypass of renal artery
L41.3   Replantation of renal artery
L41.4   Endarterectomy of renal artery
L41.5   Translocation of branch of renal artery
L41.8   Other specified
L41.9   Unspecified

L42   **Other open operations on renal artery**

L42.1   Open embolectomy of renal artery
Includes: Open thrombectomy of renal artery
Embolectomy of renal artery nec
Thrombectomy of renal artery nec
L42.2   Open embolisation of renal artery
L42.3   Ligation of renal artery
L42.4   Operations on aneurysm of renal artery
L42.8   Other specified
L42.9   Unspecified

L43   **Transluminal operations on renal artery**

L43.1   Percutaneous transluminal angioplasty of renal artery
L43.2   Percutaneous transluminal embolectomy of renal artery
Includes: Perctaneous transluminal thrombectomy of renal artery
L43.3   Percutaneous transluminal embolisation of renal artery
Includes: Embolisation of renal artery nec
L43.4   Arteriography of renal artery
L43.8   Other specified
L43.9   Unspecified

L45 **Reconstruction of other visceral branch of abdominal aorta**
Includes: Coeliac artery
Superior mesenteric artery
Inferior mesenteric artery
Suprarenal artery

L45.1 Bypass of visceral branch of abdominal aorta nec
L45.2 Replantation of visceral branch of abdominal aorta nec
L45.3 Endarterectomy of visceral branch of abdominal aorta and patch repair of visceral branch of abdominal aorta nec
L45.4 Endarterectomy of visceral branch of abdominal aorta nec
L45.8 Other specified
L45.9 Unspecified

L46 **Other open operations on other visceral branch of abdominal aorta**
Includes: Coeliac artery
Superior mesenteric artery
Inferior mesenteric artery
Suprarenal artery

L46.1 Open embolectomy of visceral branch of abdominal aorta nec
Includes: Open thrombectomy of visceral branch of abdominal aorta nec
Embolectomy of visceral branch of abdominal aorta nec
Thrombectomy of visceral branch of abdominal aorta nec
L46.2 Open embolisation of visceral branch of abdominal aorta nec
L46.3 Ligation of visceral branch of abdominal aorta nec
L46.4 Operations on aneurysm of visceral branch of abdominal aorta nec
L46.8 Other specified
L46.9 Unspecified

L47 **Transluminal operations on other visceral branch of abdominal aorta**
Includes: Coeliac artery
Superior mesenteric artery
Inferior mesenteric artery
Suprarenal artery

L47.1 Percutaneous transluminal angioplasty of visceral branch of abdominal aorta nec
L47.2 Percutaneous transluminal embolisation of visceral branch of abdominal aorta nec
Includes: Embolisation of visceral branch of abdominal aorta nec
L47.3 Arteriography of visceral branch of abdominal aorta nec
L47.8 Other specified
L47.9 Unspecified

L48   **Emergency replacement of aneurysmal iliac artery**
Includes: Emergency replacement of aneurysmal iliac artery using prosthesis
Note: *In categories L48-L54 reference to iliac artery (nfq) should be understood to include:*
common iliac artery
external iliac artery
internal iliac artery
Similarly reference to femoral artery includes:
common femoral artery
deep femoral artery
superficial femoral artery

L48.1   Emergency replacement of aneurysmal common iliac artery by anastomosis of aorta to common iliac artery

L48.2   Emergency replacement of aneurysmal iliac artery by anastomosis of aorta to external iliac artery
Includes: Emergency replacement of aneurysmal iliac artery by anastomosis of aorta to internal iliac artery

L48.3   Emergency replacement of aneurysmal artery of leg by anastomosis of aorta to common femoral artery

L48.4   Emergency replacement of aneurysmal artery of leg by anastomosis of aorta to superficial femoral artery
Includes: Emergency replacement of aneurysmal artery of leg by anastomosis of aorta to deep femoral artery
Emergency replacement of aneurysmal artery of leg by anastomosis of aorta to popliteal artery

L48.5   Emergency replacement of aneurysmal iliac artery by anastomosis of iliac artery to iliac artery

L48.6   Emergency replacement of aneurysmal artery of leg by anastomosis of iliac artery to femoral artery
Includes: Emergency replacement of aneurysmal artery of leg by anastomosis of iliac artery to popliteal artery

L48.8   Other specified
L48.9   Unspecified

L49   **Other replacement of aneurysmal iliac artery**
Note at L48 applies
Includes: Replacement of aneurysmal iliac artery using prosthesis nec

L49.1   Replacement of aneurysmal common iliac artery by anastomosis of aorta to common iliac artery nec
L49.2   Replacement of aneurysmal iliac artery by anastomosis of aorta to external iliac artery nec
Includes: Replacement of aneurysmal iliac artery by anastomosis of aorta to internal iliac artery nec
L49.3   Replacement of aneurysmal artery of leg by anastomosis of aorta to common femoral artery nec
L49.4   Replacement of aneurysmal artery of leg by anastomosis of aorta to superficial femoral artery nec
Includes: Replacement of aneurysmal artery of leg by anastomosis of aorta to deep femoral artery nec
Replacement of aneurysmal artery of leg by anastomosis of aorta to popliteal artery nec
L49.5   Replacement of aneurysmal iliac artery by anastomosis of iliac artery to iliac artery nec
L49.6   Replacement of aneurysmal artery of leg by anastomosis of iliac artery to femoral artery nec
Includes: Replacement of aneurysmal artery of leg by anastomosis of iliac artery to popliteal artery nec
L49.8   Other specified
L49.9   Unspecified

L50   **Other emergency bypass of iliac artery**
Note at L48 applies
Includes: Emergency bypass of iliac artery using prosthesis nec
Emergency replacement of iliac artery nec
Emergency replacement of iliac artery using prosthesis nec

L50.1   Emergency bypass of common iliac artery by anastomosis of aorta to common iliac artery nec
L50.2   Emergency bypass of iliac artery by anastomosis of aorta to external iliac artery nec
Includes: Emergency bypass of iliac artery by anastomosis of aorta to internal iliac artery nec
L50.3   Emergency bypass of artery of leg by anastomosis of aorta to common femoral artery nec
L50.4   Emergency bypass of artery of leg by anastomosis of aorta to deep femoral artery nec
Includes: Emergency bypass of artery of leg by anastomosis of aorta to superficial femoral artery nec
Emergency bypass of artery of leg by anastomosis of aorta to popliteal artery nec
L50.5   Emergency bypass of iliac artery by anastomosis of iliac artery to iliac artery nec
L50.6   Emergency bypass of artery of leg by anastomosis of iliac artery to femoral artery nec
Includes: Emergency bypass of artery of leg by anastomosis of iliac artery to popliteal artery nec
L50.8   Other specified
Includes: Emergency aortoiliac anastomosis nec
Emergency aortofemoral anastomosis nec
Emergency iliofemoral anastomosis nec
L50.9   Unspecified

L51   **Other bypass of iliac artery**
Note at L48 applies
Includes: Bypass of iliac artery using prosthesis nec
        Replacement of iliac artery nec
        Replacement of iliac artery using prosthesis nec

L51.1   Bypass of common iliac artery by anastomosis of aorta to common iliac artery nec
L51.2   Bypass of iliac artery by anastomosis of aorta to external iliac artery nec
        Includes: Bypass of iliac artery by anastomosis of aorta to internal iliac artery nec
L51.3   Bypass of artery of leg by anastomosis of aorta to common femoral artery nec
L51.4   Bypass of artery of leg by anastomosis of aorta to deep femoral artery nec
        Includes: Bypass of artery of leg by anastomosis of aorta to superficial femoral artery nec
        Bypass of artery of leg by anastomosis of aorta to popliteal artery nec
L51.5   Bypass of iliac artery by anastomosis of iliac artery to iliac artery nec
L51.6   Bypass of artery of leg by anastomosis of iliac artery to femoral artery nec
        Includes: Bypass of artery of leg by anastomosis of iliac artery to popliteal artery nec
L51.8   Other specified
        Includes: Aortoiliac anastomosis nec
        Aortofemoral anastomosis nec
        Iliofemoral anastomosis nec
L51.9   Unspecified

L52   **Reconstruction of iliac artery**
Note at L48 applies

L52.1   Endarterectomy of iliac artery and patch repair of iliac artery
L52.2   Endarterectomy of iliac artery nec
L52.8   Other specified
L52.9   Unspecified

L53   **Other open operations on iliac artery**
Note at L48 applies

L53.1   Repair of iliac artery nec
L53.2   Open embolectomy of iliac artery
        Includes: Open thrombectomy of iliac artery
        Embolectomy of iliac artery nec
        Thrombectomy of iliac artery nec
L53.3   Operations on aneurysm of iliac artery nec
L53.8   Other specified
L53.9   Unspecified

L54   **Transluminal operations on iliac artery**
Note at L48 applies

L54.1   Percutaneous transluminal angioplasty of iliac artery
L54.2   Percutaneous transluminal embolectomy of iliac artery
        Includes: Percutaneous transluminal thrombectomy of iliac artery
L54.3   Arteriography of iliac artery
L54.8   Other specified
L54.9   Unspecified

L56 **Emergency replacement of aneurysmal femoral artery**
Excludes: When associated with connection from aorta or iliac artery (L48)
Note: *In categories L56-L65 reference to iliac artery (nfq) should be understood to include:*
common iliac artery
external iliac artery
internal iliac artery
Similarly reference to femoral artery includes:
common femoral artery
deep femoral artery
superficial femoral artery

L56.1   Emergency replacement of aneurysmal femoral artery by anastomosis of femoral artery to femoral artery
Includes: Emergency replacement of aneurysmal femoral artery by anastomosis of femoral artery to
femoral artery using prosthesis
L56.2   Emergency replacement of aneurysmal femoral artery by anastomosis of femoral artery to popliteal artery
using prosthesis
L56.3   Emergency replacement of aneurysmal femoral artery by anastomosis of femoral artery to popliteal artery
using vein graft
Includes: Emergency replacement of aneurysmal femoral artery by anastomosis of femoral artery to
popliteal artery nec
L56.4   Emergency replacement of aneurysmal femoral artery by anastomosis of femoral artery to tibial artery
using prosthesis
Includes: Popliteal artery
L56.5   Emergency replacement of aneurysmal femoral artery by anastomosis of femoral artery to tibial artery
using vein graft
Includes: Emergency replacement of aneurysmal femoral artery by anastomosis of femoral artery to
tibial artery nec
Popliteal artery
L56.6   Emergency replacement of aneurysmal femoral artery by anastomosis of femoral artery to peroneal artery
using prosthesis
Includes: Popliteal artery
L56.7   Emergency replacement of aneurysmal femoral artery by anastomosis of femoral artery to peroneal artery
using vein graft
Includes: Emergency replacement of aneurysmal femoral artery by anastomosis of femoral artery to
peroneal artery nec
Popliteal artery
L56.8   Other specified
L56.9   Unspecified

L57   **Other replacement of aneurysmal femoral artery**
Note at L56 applies
Excludes: When associated with connection from aorta or iliac artery (L49)

L57.1   Replacement of aneurysmal femoral artery by anastomosis of femoral artery to femoral artery nec
Includes: Replacement of aneurysmal femoral artery by anastomosis of femoral artery to femoral artery using prosthesis nec

L57.2   Replacement of aneurysmal femoral artery by anastomosis of femoral artery to popliteal artery using prosthesis nec

L57.3   Replacement of aneurysmal femoral artery by anastomosis of femoral artery to popliteal artery using vein graft nec
Includes: Replacement of aneurysmal femoral artery by anastomosis of femoral artery to popliteal artery nec

L57.4   Replacement of aneurysmal femoral artery by anastomosis of femoral artery to tibial artery using prosthesis nec
Includes: Popliteal artery

L57.5   Replacement of aneurysmal femoral artery by anastomosis of femoral artery to tibial artery using vein graft nec
Includes: Replacement of aneurysmal femoral artery by anastomosis of femoral artery to tibial artery nec
Popliteal artery

L57.6   Replacement of aneurysmal femoral artery by anastomosis of femoral artery to peroneal artery using prosthesis nec
Includes: Popliteal artery

L57.7   Replacement of aneurysmal femoral artery by anastomosis of femoral artery to peroneal artery using vein graft nec
Includes: Replacement of aneurysmal femoral artery by anastomosis of femoral artery to peroneal artery nec
Popliteal artery

L57.8   Other specified
L57.9   Unspecified

L58   **Other emergency bypass of femoral artery**
Note at L56 applies
Includes: Emergency replacement of femoral artery nec
Excludes: When associated with connection from aorta or iliac artery (L50)

L58.1   Emergency bypass of femoral artery by anastomosis of femoral artery to femoral artery nec
Includes: Emergency bypass of femoral artery by anastomosis of femoral artery to femoral artery using prosthesis nec

L58.2   Emergency bypass of femoral artery by anastomosis of femoral artery to popliteal artery using prosthesis nec

L58.3   Emergency bypass of femoral artery by anastomosis of femoral artery to popliteal artery using vein graft nec
Includes: Emergency bypass of femoral artery by anastomosis of femoral artery to popliteal artery nec

L58.4   Emergency bypass of femoral artery by anastomosis of femoral artery to tibial artery using prosthesis nec
Includes: Popliteal artery

L58.5   Emergency bypass of femoral artery by anastomosis of femoral artery to tibial artery using vein graft nec
Includes: Emergency bypass of femoral artery by anastomosis of femoral artery to tibial artery nec
Popliteal artery

L58.6   Emergency bypass of femoral artery by anastomosis of femoral artery to peroneal artery using prosthesis nec
Includes: Opliteal artery

L58.7   Emergency bypass of femoral artery by anastomosis of femoral artery to peroneal artery using vein graft nec
Includes: Emergency bypass of femoral artery by anastomosis of femoral artery to peroneal artery nec
Popliteal artery

L58.8   Other specified
L58.9   Unspecified

L59 **Other bypass of femoral artery**
Note at L56 applies
Includes: Replacement of femoral artery nec
Excludes: When associated with connection from aorta or iliac artery (L51)

L59.1 Bypass of femoral artery by anastomosis of femoral artery to femoral artery nec
Includes: Bypass of femoral artery by anastomosis of femoral artery to femoral artery using prosthesis
nec
L59.2 Bypass of femoral artery by anastomosis of femoral artery to popliteal artery using prosthesis nec
L59.3 Bypass of femoral artery by anastomosis of femoral artery to popliteal artery using vein graft nec
Includes: Bypass of femoral artery by anastomosis of femoral artery to popliteal artery nec
L59.4 Bypass of femoral artery by anastomosis of femoral artery to tibial artery using prosthesis nec
Includes: Popliteal artery
L59.5 Bypass of femoral artery by anastomosis of femoral artery to tibial artery using vein graft nec
Includes: Bypass of femoral artery by anastomosis of femoral artery to tibial artery nec
Popliteal artery
L59.6 Bypass of femoral artery by anastomosis of femoral artery to peroneal artery using prosthesis nec
Includes: Popliteal artery
L59.7 Bypass of femoral artery by anastomosis of femoral artery to peroneal artery using vein graft nec
Includes: Bypass of femoral artery by anastomosis of femoral artery to peroneal artery nec
Popliteal artery
L59.8 Other specified
L59.9 Unspecified

L60 **Reconstruction of femoral artery**
Note at L56 applies
Includes: Popliteal artery

L60.1 Endarterectomy of femoral artery and patch repair of femoral artery
L60.2 Endarterectomy of femoral artery nec
L60.3 Profundoplasty of femoral artery and patch repair of deep femoral artery
L60.4 Profundoplasty of femoral artery nec
L60.8 Other specified
L60.9 Unspecified

L62 **Other open operations on femoral artery**
Note at L56 applies
Includes: Popliteal artery

L62.1 Repair of femoral artery nec
L62.2 Open embolectomy of femoral artery
Includes: Open thrombectomy of femoral artery
Embolectomy of femoral artery nec
Thrombectomy of femoral artery nec
L62.3 Ligation of aneurysm of popliteal artery
L62.4 Operations on aneurysm of femoral artery nec
L62.8 Other specified
L62.9 Unspecified

L63 **Transluminal operations on femoral artery**
Note at L56 applies
Includes: Popliteal artery

L63.1 Percutaneous transluminal angioplasty of femoral artery
L63.2 Percutaneous transluminal embolectomy of femoral artery
Includes: Percutaneous transluminal thrombectomy of femoral artery
L63.3 Percutaneous transluminal embolisation of femoral artery
Includes: Embolisation of femoral artery nec
L63.4 Arteriography of femoral artery
L63.8 Other specified
L63.9 Unspecified

L65   Revision of reconstruction of artery
Note at L56 applies

L65.1   Revision of reconstruction involving aorta
L65.2   Revision of reconstruction involving iliac artery
L65.3   Revision of reconstruction involving femoral artery
L65.8   Other specified
L65.9   Unspecified

L67   Excision of other artery
Includes: Unspecified artery
Note: These codes should not normally be used when more specific site codes may be identified (L01-L65)

L67.1   Biopsy of artery nec
L67.8   Other specified
L67.9   Unspecified

L68   Repair of other artery
Note at L67 applies
Includes: Unspecified artery

L68.1   Endarterectomy and patch repair of artery nec
L68.2   Endarterectomy nec
L68.3   Repair of artery using prosthesis nec
L68.4   Repair of artery using vein graft nec
         Includes: Repair of artery using graft nec
L68.8   Other specified
L68.9   Unspecified

L70   Other open operations on other artery
Note at L67 applies
Includes: Unspecified artery

L70.1   Open embolectomy of artery nec
         Includes: Open thrombectomy of artery nec
                 Embolectomy of artery nec
                 Thrombectomy of artery nec
L70.2   Open embolisation of artery nec
L70.3   Ligation of artery nec
L70.4   Open cannulation of artery nec
L70.5   Operations on aneurysm of artery nec
L70.8   Other specified
L70.9   Unspecified

L71   Therapeutic transluminal operations on other artery
Note at L67 applies
Includes: Unspecified artery

L71.1   Percutaneous transluminal angioplasty of artery nec
L71.2   Percutaneous transluminal embolectomy of artery nec
         Includes: Percutaneous transluminal thrombectomy of artery nec
L71.3   Percutaneous transluminal embolisation of artery nec
         Includes: Embolisation of artery nec
L71.4   Percutaneous transluminal cannulation of artery nec
         Includes: Cannulation of artery nec
L71.5   Percutaneous transluminal dilation of artery nec
L71.8   Other specified
L71.9   Unspecified

L72 **Diagnostic transluminal operations on other artery**
Note at L67 applies
Includes: Unspecified artery

L72.1 Arteriography nec
L72.2 Monitoring of arterial pressure
L72.3 Percutaneous transluminal angioscopy nec
L72.8 Other specified
L72.9 Unspecified

L74 **Arteriovenous shunt**

L74.1 Insertion of arteriovenous prosthesis
L74.2 Creation of arteriovenous fistula nec
L74.3 Attention to arteriovenous shunt
L74.8 Other specified
L74.9 Unspecified

L75 **Other arteriovenous operations**

L75.1 Excision of congenital arteriovenous malformation
Includes: Ligation of congenital arteriovenous malformation
L75.2 Repair of acquired arteriovenous fistula
Includes: Ligation of acquired arteriovenous fistula
L75.3 Embolisation of arteriovenous abnormality
L75.8 Other specified
L75.9 Unspecified

L77 **Connection of vena cava or branch of vena cava**

L77.1 Creation of portocaval shunt
L77.2 Creation of mesocaval shunt
L77.3 Creation of portosystemic shunt nec
L77.4 Creation of distal splenorenal shunt
L77.5 Creation of proximal splenorenal shunt
L77.8 Other specified
L77.9 Unspecified

L79 **Other operations on vena cava**

L79.1 Insertion of filter into vena cava
L79.2 Plication of vena cava
L79.8 Other specified
L79.9 Unspecified

L81 **Other bypass operations on vein**

L81.1 Creation of peritovenous shunt
L81.2 Bypass operations for priapism
L81.8 Other specified
L81.9 Unspecified

L82 **Repair of valve of vein**

L82.1 Transposition of valve of vein
L82.2 Interposition of valve of vein
L82.8 Other specified
L82.9 Unspecified

L83 **Other operations for venous insufficiency**

L83.1 Crossover graft of saphenous vein
L83.2 Subfascial ligation of perforating vein of leg
L83.8 Other specified
L83.9 Unspecified

L85 **Ligation of varicose vein of leg**

L85.1 Ligation of long saphenous vein
L85.2 Ligation of short saphenous vein
L85.3 Ligation of recurrent varicose vein of leg
L85.8 Other specified
L85.9 Unspecified

L86 **Injection into varicose vein of leg**

L86.1 Injection of sclerosing substance into varicose vein of leg
L86.8 Other specified
L86.9 Unspecified

L87 **Other operations on varicose vein of leg**

L87.1 Stripping of long saphenous vein
L87.2 Stripping of short saphenous vein
L87.3 Stripping of varicose vein of leg nec
L87.4 Avulsion of varicose vein of leg
L87.5 Local excision of varicose vein of leg
L87.6 Incision of varicose vein of leg
L87.8 Other specified
L87.9 Unspecified

L90 **Open removal of thrombus from vein**

L90.1 Open thrombectomy of vein of upper limb
L90.2 Open thrombectomy of vein of lower limb
L90.8 Other specified
L90.9 Unspecified

L91 **Other vein related operations**

L91.1 Open insertion of central venous catheter
L91.2 Insertion of central venous catheter nec
L91.3 Attention to central venous catheter
L91.8 Other specified
L91.9 Unspecified

L93 **Other open operations on vein**
       Excludes: Operations on varicocele (N19)

L93.1 Excision of vein nec
       Includes: Biopsy of vein
L93.2 Incision of vein nec
L93.3 Ligation of vein nec
L93.4 Open cannulation of vein
L93.8 Other specified
L93.9 Unspecified

L94 **Therapeutic transluminal operations on vein**

L94.1 Percutaneous transluminal embolisation of vein
L94.2 Percutaneous transluminal cannulation of vein
L94.8 Other specified
L94.9 Unspecified

L95 **Diagnostic transluminal operations on vein**

L95.1 Venography
L95.8 Other specified
L95.9 Unspecified

L97 Other operations on blood vessel

L97.1 Revascularisation for impotence
L97.2 Peroperative angioplasty
L97.3 Isolated limb perfusion
L97.4 Operations on artery nec
L97.5 Operations on vein nec
L97.8 Other specified
L97.9 Unspecified

CHAPTER M

URINARY

(CODES M01-M83)

Includes: PROSTATE

Excludes: PENIS (except URETHRAL ORIFICE)   (Chapter N)
OPERATIONS FOR SEXUAL TRANSFORMATION   (Chapter X)

M01   **Transplantation of kidney**

M01.1   Autotransplantation of kidney
M01.2   Allotransplantation of kidney from live donor
M01.3   Allotransplantation of kidney from cadaver
M01.8   Other specified
M01.9   Unspecified

M02   **Total excision of kidney**

M02.1   Nephrectomy and excision of perirenal tissue
      Includes: Nephroureterectomy and excision of perirenal tissue
M02.2   Nephroureterectomy nec
M02.3   Bilateral nephrectomy
M02.4   Excision of half of horseshoe kidney
M02.5   Nephrectomy nec
M02.6   Excision of rejected transplanted kidney
M02.8   Other specified
M02.9   Unspecified

M03   **Partial excision of kidney**

M03.1   Heminephrectomy of duplex kidney
M03.2   Division of isthmus of horseshoe kidney
M03.8   Other specified
M03.9   Unspecified
      Includes: Partial nephrectomy nec

M04   **Open extirpation of lesion of kidney**

M04.1   Deroofing of cyst of kidney
M04.2   Open excision of lesion of kidney nec
M04.3   Open destruction of lesion of kidney
M04.8   Other specified
M04.9   Unspecified

M05   **Open repair of kidney**

M05.1   Open pyeloplasty
M05.2   Open revision of pyeloplasty
M05.3   Nephropexy
M05.4   Plication of kidney
      Note: *Use additional code for coincidental translocation of branch of renal artery (L41.5)*
M05.5   Repair of laceration of kidney
M05.8   Other specified
M05.9   Unspecified

M06   **Incision of kidney**
Includes: Pelvis of kidney

M06.1   Open removal of calculus from kidney
Includes: Nephrolithotomy
                Pyelolithotomy
M06.2   Drainage of kidney nec
Includes: Nephrostomy nec
                Insertion of nephrostomy tube
M06.3   Closure of nephrostomy
M06.8   Other specified
M06.9   Unspecified

M08   **Other open operations on kidney**
Includes: Pelvis of kidney

M08.1   Open biopsy of lesion of kidney
Includes: Open biopsy of kidney
M08.2   Open denervation of kidney
M08.3   Exploration of kidney
M08.4   Exploration of transplanted kidney
M08.8   Other specified
M08.9   Unspecified

M09   **Therapeutic endoscopic operations on calculus of kidney**
Includes: Nephroscopic percutaneous lithotripsy of calculus of kidney
Percutaneous lithotripsy of calculus of kidney nec
Note: It is not necessary to code additionally any mention of diagnostic endoscopic examination of kidney (M11.9)

M09.1   Endoscopic ultrasound fragmentation of calculus of kidney
M09.2   Endoscopic electrohydraulic shock wave fragmentation of calculus of kidney
M09.3   Endoscopic laser fragmentation of calculus of kidney
M09.4   Endoscopic extraction of calculus of kidney nec
M09.8   Other specified
M09.9   Unspecified

M10   **Other therapeutic endoscopic operations on kidney**
Note: It is not necessary to code additionally any mention of diagnostic endoscopic examination of kidney (M11.9)

M10.1   Endoscopic extirpation of lesion of kidney
M10.2   Endoscopic pyeloplasty
M10.8   Other specified
M10.9   Unspecified

M11   **Diagnostic endoscopic examination of kidney**

M11.1   Diagnostic endoscopic examination of kidney and biopsy of lesion of kidney
Includes: Diagnostic endoscopic examination of kidney and biopsy of kidney
                Endoscopic biopsy of lesion of kidney
                Endoscopic biopsy of kidney
M11.8   Other specified
M11.9   Unspecified
Includes: Nephroscopy nec

M13　**Percutaneous puncture of kidney**
Includes: Pelvis of kidney
Note:　Use subsidiary code to identify method of image control as necessary (Y53)

M13.1　Percutaneous needle biopsy of lesion of kidney
Includes: Percutaneous needle biopsy of kidney
Biopsy of lesion of kidney nec
Biopsy of kidney nec
M13.2　Percutaneous drainage of kidney
M13.3　Percutaneous aspiration of kidney nec
M13.4　Percutaneous injection of therapeutic substance into kidney
M13.5　Percutaneous injection of radiocontrast substance into kidney
Includes: Antegrade pyelography
M13.6　Percutaneous insertion of nephrostomy tube
M13.8　Other specified
M13.9　Unspecified

M14　**Extracorporeal fragmentation of calculus of kidney**

M14.1　Extracorporeal shock wave lithotripsy of calculus of kidney
M14.8　Other specified
M14.9　Unspecified

M15　**Operations on kidney along nephrostomy tube track**

M15.1　Nephrostomography
M15.8　Other specified
M15.9　Unspecified

M16　**Other operations on kidney**
Excludes: Renal dialysis (X40.1)

M16.1　Irrigation of kidney
M16.2　Maintenance of drainage tube of kidney
Includes: Maintenance of nephrostomy tube
M16.8　Other specified
M16.9　Unspecified

M18　**Excision of ureter**

M18.1　Total ureterectomy
Includes: Ureterectomy nec
M18.2　Excision of segment of ureter
M18.3　Secondary ureterectomy
M18.8　Other specified
M18.9　Unspecified

M19　**Urinary diversion**

M19.1　Construction of ileal conduit
M19.2　Creation of urinary diversion to intestine nec
M19.3　Revision of urinary diversion
Includes: Revision of ileal conduit
M19.4　Cutaneous ureterostomy nec
M19.5　Revision of ureterostomy stoma
M19.8　Other specified
M19.9　Unspecified

M20　**Replantation of ureter**

M20.1　Bilateral replantation of ureter
M20.2　Unilateral replantation of ureter
M20.3　Replantation of ureter after urinary diversion
M20.8　Other specified
M20.9　Unspecified

M21   Other connection of ureter

M21.1   Direct anastomosis of ureter to bladder
M21.2   Anastomosis of ureter to bladder using flap of bladder
M21.3   Ileal replacement of ureter
M21.4   Colonic replacement of ureter
M21.5   Revision of anastomosis of ureter nec
M21.8   Other specified
M21.9   Unspecified

M22   Repair of ureter

M22.1   Suture of ureter
M22.2   Removal of ligature from ureter
M22.8   Other specified
M22.9   Unspecified

M23   Incision of ureter

M23.1   Open ureterolithotomy
M23.8   Other specified
M23.9   Unspecified

M25   Other open operations on ureter

M25.1   Excision of ureterocele
M25.2   Open excision of lesion of ureter nec
M25.3   Ureterolysis
M25.4   Open biopsy of lesion of ureter
         Includes: Open biopsy of ureter
M25.8   Other specified
M25.9   Unspecified

M26   Therapeutic nephroscopic operations on ureter
         Note: It is not necessary to code additionally any mention of diagnostic endoscopic examination of ureter (M30.9)

M26.1   Nephroscopic laser fragmentation of calculus of ureter
M26.2   Nephroscopic fragmentation of calculus of ureter nec
M26.3   Nephroscopic extraction of calculus of ureter
M26.4   Nephroscopic insertion of tubal prosthesis into ureter
M26.8   Other specified
M26.9   Unspecified

M27   Therapeutic ureteroscopic operations on ureter
         Note: It is not necessary to code additionally any mention of diagnostic endoscopic examination of ureter (M30.9)

M27.1   Ureteroscopic laser fragmentation of calculus of ureter
M27.2   Ureteroscopic fragmentation of calculus of ureter nec
M27.3   Ureteroscopic extraction of calculus of ureter
M27.8   Other specified
M27.9   Unspecified

M28   Other endoscopic removal of calculus from ureter
         Includes: Cystoscopic removal of calculus from ureter
         Note: It is not necessary to code additionally any mention of diagnostic endoscopic examination of ureter (M30.9)

M28.1   Endoscopic laser fragmentation of calculus of ureter nec
M28.2   Endoscopic fragmentation of calculus of ureter nec
M28.3   Endoscopic extraction of calculus of ureter nec
M28.4   Endoscopic catheter drainage of calculus of ureter
M28.5   Endoscopic drainage of calculus of ureter by dilation of ureter
M28.8   Other specified
M28.9   Unspecified

M29   **Other therapeutic endoscopic operations on ureter**
Includes: Therapeutic cystoscopic operations on ureter nec
Note: *It is not necessary to code additionally any mention of diagnostic endoscopic examination of ureter (M30.9)*

M29.1   Endoscopic extirpation of lesion of ureter
M29.2   Endoscopic insertion of tubal prosthesis into ureter nec
M29.3   Endoscopic removal of tubal prosthesis from ureter
M29.4   Endoscopic dilation of ureter
M29.8   Other specified
M29.9   Unspecified

M30   **Diagnostic endoscopic examination of ureter**
Includes: Diagnostic cystoscopic examination of ureter
Note: *Use as supplementary code when associated with diagnostic endoscopic examination of bladder (M45)*

M30.1   Endoscopic retrograde pyelography
M30.2   Endoscopic catheterisation of ureter
M30.8   Other specified
M30.9   Unspecified
Includes: Ureteroscopy nec

M31   **Extracorporeal fragmentation of calculus of ureter**

M31.1   Extracorporeal shockwave lithotripsy of calculus of ureter
M31.8   Other specified
M31.9   Unspecified

M32   **Operations on ureteric orifice**
Note: *It is not necessary to code additionally any mention of diagnostic endoscopic examination of ureter (M30.9)*

M32.1   Endoscopic extirpation of lesion of ureteric orifice
M32.2   Endoscopic meatotomy of ureteric orifice
M32.3   Endoscopic injection of inert substance around ureteric orifice
M32.8   Other specified
M32.9   Unspecified

M34   **Total excision of bladder**

M34.1   Cystoprostatectomy
M34.2   Cystourethrectomy
M34.3   Cystectomy nec
M34.4   Simple cystectomy
M34.8   Other specified
M34.9   Unspecified

M35   **Partial excision of bladder**

M35.1   Diverticulectomy of bladder
M35.8   Other specified
M35.9   Unspecified
Includes: Partial cystectomy nec

M36   **Enlargement of bladder**

M36.1   Caecocystoplasty
M36.2   Ileocystoplasty
M36.3   Colocystoplasty
M36.8   Other specified
M36.9   Unspecified

M37   Other repair of bladder

M37.1   Cystourethroplasty
M37.2   Repair of vesicocolic fistula
M37.3   Repair of rupture of bladder
M37.8   Other specified
M37.9   Unspecified

M38   Open drainage of bladder

M38.1   Perineal urethrostomy and drainage of bladder
M38.2   Cystostomy and insertion of suprapubic tube into bladder
M38.8   Other specified
M38.9   Unspecified

M39   Other open operations on contents of bladder

M39.1   Open removal of calculus from bladder
M39.2   Open removal of foreign body from bladder
M39.8   Other specified
M39.9   Unspecified

M41   Other open operations on bladder

M41.1   Open extirpation of lesion of bladder
M41.2   Creation of vesicovaginal fistula
M41.3   Open transection of bladder
M41.4   Open biopsy of lesion of bladder
        Includes: Open biopsy of bladder
M41.5   Exploration of bladder
M41.8   Other specified
M41.9   Unspecified

M42   Endoscopic extirpation of lesion of bladder
        *Note: It is not necessary to code additionally any mention of diagnostic endoscopic examination of
                  bladder (M45.9)*

M42.1   Endoscopic resection of lesion of bladder
M42.2   Endoscopic cauterisation of lesion of bladder
M42.3   Endoscopic destruction of lesion of bladder nec
M42.8   Other specified
M42.9   Unspecified

M43   Endoscopic operations to increase capacity of bladder
        *Note: It is not necessary to code additionally any mention of diagnostic endoscopic examination of
                  bladder (M45.9)*

M43.1   Endoscopic transection of bladder
M43.2   Endoscopic hydrostatic distention of bladder
M43.3   Endoscopic overdistention of bladder nec
M43.4   Endoscopic injection of neurolytic substance into nerve of bladder
M43.8   Other specified
M43.9   Unspecified

M44   Other therapeutic endoscopic operations on bladder
        *Note: It is not necessary to code additionally any mention of diagnostic endoscopic examination of
                  bladder (M45.9)*

M44.1   Endoscopic lithopaxy
M44.2   Endoscopic extraction of calculus of bladder nec
M44.3   Endoscopic removal of foreign body from bladder
M44.4   Endoscopic removal of blood clot from bladder
M44.8   Other specified
M44.9   Unspecified

M45 **Diagnostic endoscopic examination of bladder**
Includes: Prostate (M45.2)
Note: *Use supplementary code for diagnostic endoscopic examination of ureter (M30)*

M45.1 Diagnostic endoscopic examination of bladder and biopsy of lesion of bladder
Includes: Diagnostic endoscopic examination of bladder and biopsy of bladder
Endoscopic biopsy of lesion of bladder
Endoscopic biopsy of bladder
Biopsy of lesion of bladder nec
Biopsy of bladder nec
M45.2 Diagnostic endoscopic examination of bladder and biopsy of lesion of prostate
Includes: Diagnostic endoscopic examination of bladder and biopsy of prostate
Endoscopic biopsy of lesion of prostate
Endoscopic biopsy of prostate
M45.8 Other specified
M45.9 Unspecified
Includes: Cystourethroscopy nec
Cystoscopy nec

M47 **Urethral catheterisation of bladder**

M47.1 Urethral irrigation of bladder
Includes: Urethral lavage of bladder
M47.2 Change of urethral catheter into bladder
M47.3 Removal of urethral catheter from bladder
M47.8 Other specified
M47.9 Unspecified

M49 **Other operations on bladder**

M49.1 Closure of cystostomy
M49.2 Change of suprapubic tube into bladder
M49.3 Removal of suprapubic tube from bladder
M49.4 Introduction of therapeutic substance into bladder
M49.8 Other specified
M49.9 Unspecified

M51 **Combined abdominal and vaginal operations to support outlet of female bladder**

M51.1 Abdominoperineal suspension of urethra
Includes: Abdominovaginal suspension of urethra
M51.2 Endoscopic suspension of neck of bladder
M51.8 Other specified
M51.9 Unspecified

M52 **Abdominal operations to support outlet of female bladder**

M52.1 Suprapubic sling operation
M52.2 Retropubic suspension of neck of bladder
M52.3 Colposuspension of neck of bladder
M52.4 Urethrolysis
M52.8 Other specified
M52.9 Unspecified

M53 **Vaginal operations to support outlet of female bladder**

M53.1 Vaginal buttressing of urethra
M53.2 Introduction of biethium bean through vagina
M53.8 Other specified
M53.9 Unspecified

M55   Other open operations on outlet of female bladder

M55.1   Open resection of outlet of female bladder
M55.2   Implantation of artificial urinary sphincter into outlet of female bladder
M55.3   Insertion of prosthetic collar around outlet of female bladder
M55.4   Maintenance of prosthetic collar around outlet of female bladder
M55.5   Removal of prosthetic collar from around outlet of female bladder
M55.8   Other specified
M55.9   Unspecified

M56   Therapeutic endoscopic operations on outlet of female bladder
Note: It is not necessary to code additionally any mention of diagnostic endoscopic examination of bladder (M45.9)

M56.1   Endoscopic resection of outlet of female bladder
M56.2   Endoscopic incision of outlet of female bladder
M56.3   Endoscopic injection of inert substance into outlet of female bladder
M56.8   Other specified
M56.9   Unspecified

M58   Other operations on outlet of female bladder

M58.1   Closed urethrotomy of outlet of female bladder
M58.2   Dilation of outlet of female bladder
M58.8   Other specified
M58.9   Unspecified

M61   Open excision of prostate
Excludes: Cystoprostatectomy (M34.1)

M61.1   Total excision of prostate and capsule of prostate
M61.2   Retropubic prostatectomy
M61.3   Transvesical prostatectomy
M61.4   Perineal prostatectomy
M61.8   Other specified
M61.9   Unspecified
         Includes: Prostatectomy nec

M62   Other open operations on prostate

M62.1   Open extirpation of lesion of prostate
M62.2   Open biopsy of lesion of prostate
         Includes: Open biopsy of prostate
M62.3   Prostatotomy
M62.8   Other specified
M62.9   Unspecified

M64   Other open operations on outlet of male bladder

M64.1   Open resection of outlet of male bladder
M64.2   Implantation of artificial urinary sphincter into outlet of male bladder
M64.3   Insertion of prosthetic collar around outlet of male bladder
M64.4   Maintenance of prosthetic collar around outlet of male bladder
M64.5   Removal of prosthetic collar from around outlet of male bladder
M64.8   Other specified
M64.9   Unspecified

M65 **Endoscopic resection of outlet of male bladder**
Includes: Endoscopic resection of lesion of outlet of male bladder
Note: *It is not necessary to code additionally any mention of diagnostic endoscopic examination of bladder (M45.9)*

M65.1 Endoscopic resection of prostate using electrotome
M65.2 Endoscopic resection of prostate using punch
M65.3 Endoscopic resection of prostate nec
M65.8 Other specified
M65.9 Unspecified

M66 **Other therapeutic endoscopic operations on outlet of male bladder**
Note: *It is not necessary to code additionally any mention of diagnostic endoscopic examination of bladder (M45.9)*

M66.1 Endoscopic sphincterotomy of external sphincter of male bladder
M66.2 Endoscopic incision of outlet of male bladder nec
M66.3 Endoscopic injection of inert substance into outlet of male bladder
M66.8 Other specified
M66.9 Unspecified

M67 **Other therapeutic endoscopic operations on prostate**
Note: *It is not necessary to code additionally any mention of diagnostic endoscopic examination of bladder (M45.9)*

M67.1 Endoscopic cryotherapy to lesion of prostate
M67.2 Endoscopic destruction of lesion of prostate nec
M67.3 Endoscopic drainage of prostate
M67.4 Endoscopic removal of calculus from prostate
M67.8 Other specified
M67.9 Unspecified

M70 **Other operations on outlet of male bladder**

M70.1 Aspiration of prostate nec
M70.2 Perineal needle biopsy of prostate
Includes: Needle biopsy of prostate nec
Biopsy of prostate nec
M70.3 Rectal needle biopsy of prostate
M70.4 Balloon dilation of prostate
M70.5 Massage of prostate
M70.8 Other specified
M70.9 Unspecified

M72 **Excision of urethra**

M72.1 Partial urethrectomy
M72.2 Urethrectomy nec
M72.3 Excision of lesion of urethra nec
M72.8 Other specified
M72.9 Unspecified

M73 **Repair of urethra**

M73.1 Repair of hypospadias
M73.2 Repair of epispadias
M73.3 Closure of fistula of urethra
M73.4 Reconstruction of urethra
M73.5 Pull through of urethra
M73.6 Urethroplasty nec
M73.8 Other specified
M73.9 Unspecified

M75 Other open operations on urethra

M75.1 Open biopsy of lesion of urethra
Includes: Open biopsy of urethra
M75.2 Insertion of prosthesis for compression of bulb of male urethra
M75.3 External urethrotomy
Note: Do not use as approach code (Y52.2)
M75.8 Other specified
M75.9 Unspecified

M76 Therapeutic endoscopic operations on urethra
Note: It is not necessary to code additionally any mention of diagnostic endoscopic examination of urethra (M77.9)

M76.1 Endoscopic extirpation of lesion of urethra
M76.2 Endoscopic removal of foreign body from urethra
M76.3 Optical urethrotomy
M76.4 Endoscopic dilation of urethra
M76.8 Other specified
M76.9 Unspecified

M77 Diagnostic endoscopic examination of urethra

M77.1 Diagnostic endoscopic examination of urethra and biopsy of lesion of urethra
Includes: Diagnostic endoscopic examination of urethra and biopsy of urethra
Endoscopic biopsy of lesion of urethra
Endoscopic biopsy of urethra
Biopsy of lesion of urethra nec
Biopsy of urethra nec
M77.8 Other specified
M77.9 Unspecified
Includes: Urethroscopy nec

M79 Other operations on urethra

M79.1 Bouginage of urethra
M79.2 Dilation of urethra nec
M79.3 Calibration of urethra
M79.4 Internal urethrotomy nec
M79.8 Other specified
M79.9 Unspecified

M81 Operations on urethral orifice

M81.1 Extirpation of lesion of meatus of urethra
M81.2 Meatoplasty of urethra
M81.3 External meatotomy of urethral orifice
M81.4 Dilation of meatus of urethra
M81.8 Other specified
M81.9 Unspecified

M83 Other operations on urinary tract

M83.1 Drainage of paravesical abscess
M83.2 Exploration of retropubic space
M83.3 Removal of foreign body from urinary tract nec
M83.8 Other specified
M83.9 Unspecified

CHAPTER N

MALE GENITAL ORGANS

(CODES N01-N34)

Excludes: PROSTATE   (Chapter M)
         URETHRAL ORIFICE   (Chapter M)
         OPERATIONS FOR MALE
         SEXUAL TRANSFORMATION   (Chapter X)

N01   **Extirpation of scrotum**
Includes: Skin of scrotum
Note: Codes from Chapter S may be used to enhance these codes

N01.1   Excision of scrotum
N01.2   Excision of lesion of scrotum
N01.3   Destruction of lesion of scrotum
N01.8   Other specified
N01.9   Unspecified

N03   **Other operations on scrotum**
Note at N01 applies
Includes: Skin of scrotum

N03.1   Biopsy of lesion of scrotum
        Includes: Biopsy of scrotum
N03.2   Drainage of scrotum
N03.3   Suture of scrotum
N03.4   Exploration of scrotum
N03.8   Other specified
N03.9   Unspecified

N05   **Bilateral excision of testes**

N05.1   Bilateral subcapsular orchidectomy
N05.2   Bilateral orchidectomy nec
N05.8   Other specified
N05.9   Unspecified
        Includes: Male castration

N06   **Other excision of testis**

N06.1   Subcapsular orchidectomy nec
N06.2   Excision of aberrant testis
N06.3   Orchidectomy nec
N06.8   Other specified
N06.9   Unspecified

N07   **Extirpation of lesion of testis**

N07.1   Excision of lesion of testis
N07.2   Destruction of lesion of testis
N07.8   Other specified
N07.9   Unspecified

N08   **Bilateral placement of testes in scrotum**

N08.1   Bilateral microvascular transfer of testes to scrotum
N08.2   One stage bilateral orchidopexy nec
N08.3   First stage bilateral orchidopexy
N08.4   Second stage bilateral orchidopexy
N08.8   Other specified
N08.9   Unspecified

N09   **Other placement of testis in scrotum**

N09.1   Microvascular transfer of testis to scrotum nec
N09.2   One stage orchidopexy nec
N09.3   First stage orchidopexy nec
N09.4   Second stage orchidopexy nec
N09.8   Other specified
N09.9   Unspecified

N10   **Prosthesis of testis**

N10.1   Insertion of prosthetic replacement for testis
N10.2   Removal of prosthetic replacement for testis
N10.8   Other specified
N10.9   Unspecified

N11   **Operations on hydrocele sac**
          Excludes: Correction of hydrocele of infancy (T19.3)

N11.1   Excision of hydrocele sac
N11.2   Plication of hydrocele sac
N11.3   Eversion of hydrocele sac
N11.4   Drainage of hydrocele sac
N11.5   Aspiration of hydrocele sac
          Includes: Tapping of hydrocele sac
N11.6   Injection sclerotherapy to hydrocele sac
N11.8   Other specified
N11.9   Unspecified

N13   **Other operations on testis**

N13.1   Drainage of testis
N13.2   Fixation of testis
          Includes: Tether of testis
N13.3   Reduction of torsion of testis
N13.4   Biopsy of testis
          Includes: Biopsy of lesion of testis
N13.5   Exploration of testis
N13.8   Other specified
N13.9   Unspecified

N15   **Operations on epididymis**

N15.1   Bilateral epididymectomy
N15.2   Unilateral epididymectomy
N15.3   Excision of lesion of epididymis
N15.4   Drainage of epididymis
N15.5   Biopsy of lesion of epididymis
          Includes: Biopsy of epididymis
N15.6   Aspiration of lesion of epididymis
N15.7   Epididymovasostomy
N15.8   Other specified
N15.9   Unspecified
          Includes: Epididymectomy nec

N17 Excision of vas deferens

N17.1 Bilateral vasectomy
Includes: Vasectomy nec
N17.2 Ligation of vas deferens nec
N17.8 Other specified
N17.9 Unspecified

N18 Repair of spermatic cord

N18.1 Reversal of bilateral vasectomy
N18.2 Suture of vas deferens nec
N18.8 Other specified
N18.9 Unspecified

N19 Operations on varicocele

N19.1 Ligation of varicocele
N19.2 Embolisation of varicocele
N19.8 Other specified
N19.9 Unspecified

N20 Other operations on spermatic cord

N20.1 Excision of lesion of spermatic cord
N20.2 Biopsy of spermatic cord
Includes: Biopsy of lesion of spermatic cord
N20.3 Drainage of spermatic cord
N20.4 Vasotomy
N20.5 Vasography
N20.8 Other specified
N20.9 Unspecified

N22 Operations on seminal vesicle

N22.1 Excision of seminal vesicle
N22.2 Incision of seminal vesicle
N22.3 Seminal vesiculography
N22.8 Other specified
N22.9 Unspecified

N24 Operations on male perineum
Includes: Skin of male perineun (N24.1 N24.2)
Note: Codes from Chapter S may be used to enhance these codes

N24.1 Excision of sweat gland bearing skin of male perineum
N24.2 Operations on skin of male perineum nec
N24.3 Excision of male periurethral tissue nec
N24.4 Incision of male periurethral tissue
N24.8 Other specified
N24.9 Unspecified

N26 Amputation of penis

N26.1 Total amputation of penis
N26.2 Partial amputation of penis
N26.8 Other specified
N26.9 Unspecified

N27 **Extirpation of lesion of penis**
Includes: Skin of penis
Note: *Codes from Chapter S may be used to enhance these codes*

N27.1 Excision of lesion of penis
N27.2 Cauterisation of lesion of penis
N27.3 Destruction of lesion of penis nec
N27.8 Other specified
N27.9 Unspecified

N28 **Plastic operations on penis**
Note at N27 applies
Includes: Skin of penis

N28.1 Construction of penis
N28.2 Reconstruction of penis
N28.3 Plication of corpora of penis
N28.4 Frenuloplasty of penis
N28.5 Correction of chordee of penis
N28.8 Other specified
N28.9 Unspecified

N29 **Prosthesis of penis**

N29.1 Implantation of prosthesis into penis
N29.2 Attention to prosthesis in penis
N29.8 Other specified
N29.9 Unspecified

N30 **Operations on prepuce**
Includes: Skin of prepuce
Note: *Codes from Chapter S may be used to enhance these codes*

N30.1 Prepuceplasty
N30.2 Freeing of adhesions of prepuce
N30.3 Circumcision
N30.4 Dorsal slit of prepuce
Includes: Lateral slit of prepuce
N30.5 Stretching of prepuce
N30.6 Manual reduction of prepuce
N30.8 Other specified
N30.9 Unspecified

N32 **Other operations on penis**
Note at N27 applies
Includes: Skin of penis

N32.1 Biopsy of lesion of penis
Includes: Biopsy of penis
N32.2 Drainage of penis
N32.3 Incision of penis nec
N32.8 Other specified
N32.9 Unspecified

N34 **Other operations on male genital tract**

N34.1 Fertility investigation of male nec
N34.2 Collection of sperm
N34.3 Male colposcopy
N34.8 Other specified
N34.9 Unspecified

CHAPTER P

LOWER FEMALE GENITAL TRACT

(CODES P01-P31)

Excludes: GYNAECOLOGICAL OPERATIONS ON
        FEMALE URETHRA AND BLADDER   (Chapter M)
        OBSTETRIC OPERATIONS   (Chapter R)
        OPERATIONS FOR FEMALE
        SEXUAL TRANSFORMATION   (Chapter X)

Note: *Obstetric operations are normally carried out in relation to delivery at or near term or in pregnancy expected to go to term They do not include abortion or termination of pregnancy*

P01	**Operations on clitoris**
P01.1	Clitoridectomy
P01.8	Other specified
P01.9	Unspecified

P03   **Operations on Bartholin gland**
            Includes: Bartholin duct (P03.5)

P03.1	Excision of Bartholin gland
P03.2	Marsupialisation of Bartholin gland
P03.3	Excision of lesion of Bartholin gland
P03.4	Drainage of Bartholin gland
P03.5	Operations on Bartholin duct
P03.8	Other specified
P03.9	Unspecified

P05   **Excision of vulva**
            Includes: Skin of vulva
            Note: *Codes from Chapter S may be used to enhance these codes*

P05.1	Total excision of vulva
P05.2	Partial excision of vulva
P05.3	Marsupialisation of lesion of vulva
P05.4	Excision of lesion of vulva nec
P05.5	Excision of excess labial tissue
P05.8	Other specified
P05.9	Unspecified

            Includes: Vulvectomy nec

P06   **Extirpation of lesion of vulva**
            Note at P05 applies
            Includes: Skin of vulva

P06.1	Laser destruction of lesion of vulva
P06.2	Cryosurgery to lesion of vulva
P06.3	Cauterisation of lesion of vulva
P06.4	Implantation of radioactive substance into vulva
P06.8	Other specified
P06.9	Unspecified

P07 **Repair of vulva**
Note at P05 applies
Includes: Skin of vulva

P07.1 Plastic repair of vulva
P07.8 Other specified
P07.9 Unspecified

P09 **Other operations on vulva**
Note at P05 applies
Includes: Skin of vulva

P09.1 Biopsy of lesion of vulva
Includes: Biopsy of vulva
P09.2 Drainage of lesion of vulva
P09.3 Evacuation of haematoma from vulva
P09.8 Other specified
P09.9 Unspecified

P11 **Extirpation of lesion of female perineum**
Includes: Skin of female perineum
Note: Codes from Chapter S may be used to enhance these codes

P11.1 Excision of lesion of female perineum
P11.2 Laser destruction of lesion of female perineum
P11.3 Cauterisation of lesion of female perineum
P11.4 Destruction of lesion of female perineum nec
P11.8 Other specified
P11.9 Unspecified

P13 **Other operations on female perineum**
Note at P11 applies
Includes: Skin of female perineum

P13.1 Drainage of female perineum
Includes: Drainage of lesion of female perineum
P13.2 Female perineorrhaphy
Excludes: Colpoperineorrhaphy (P25.5)
P13.3 Female perineoplasty
P13.4 Closure of fistula of female perineum
P13.5 Female perineotomy nec
P13.6 Operations on female periurethral tissue nec
P13.7 Excision of sweat gland bearing skin of female perineum
P13.8 Other specified
P13.9 Unspecified

P14 **Incision of introitus of vagina**

P14.1 Posterior episiotomy and division of levator ani muscle
P14.2 Posterior episiotomy nec
P14.3 Anterior episiotomy
P14.8 Other specified
P14.9 Unspecified
Includes: Episiotomy nec

P15 **Other operations on introitus of vagina**

P15.1 Hymenectomy
P15.2 Excision of hymenal tag
P15.3 Repair of hymen
P15.4 Incision of hymen
Includes: Hymenotomy
P15.5 Stretching of hymen
P15.8 Other specified
P15.9 Unspecified

P17   **Excision of vagina**

P17.1   Total colpectomy
P17.2   Partial colpectomy
P17.3   Marsupialisation of lesion of vagina
P17.8   Other specified
P17.9   Unspecified

P18   **Other obliteration of vagina**

P18.1   Complete colpocleisis
P18.2   Partial colpocleisis
P18.8   Other specified
P18.9   Unspecified

P19   **Excision of band of vagina**

P19.1   Laser excision of septum of vagina
P19.2   Excision of septum of vagina nec
P19.8   Other specified
P19.9   Unspecified

P20   **Extirpation of lesion of vagina**

P20.1   Excision of lesion of vagina
P20.2   Laser destruction of lesion of vagina
P20.3   Cauterisation of lesion of vagina
P20.4   Cryotherapy to lesion of vagina
P20.5   Implantation of radioactive substance into vagina
P20.8   Other specified
P20.9   Unspecified

P21   **Plastic operations on vagina**

P21.1   Construction of vagina
P21.2   Reconstruction of vagina
P21.3   Vaginoplasty nec
P21.8   Other specified
P21.9   Unspecified

P22   **Repair of prolapse of vagina and amputation of cervix uteri**

P22.1   Anterior and posterior colporrhaphy and amputation of cervix uteri
P22.2   Anterior colporrhaphy and amputation of cervix uteri nec
P22.3   Posterior colporrhaphy and amputation of cervix uteri nec
P22.8   Other specified
P22.9   Unspecified
        Includes: Colporrhaphy and amputation of cervix uteri nec

P23   **Other repair of prolapse of vagina**
        Note: *Use supplementary code for concurrent excision of uterus (Q08)*

P23.1   Anterior and posterior colporrhaphy nec
P23.2   Anterior colporrhaphy nec
P23.3   Posterior colporrhaphy nec
P23.4   Repair of enterocele nec
P23.8   Other specified
P23.9   Unspecified
        Includes: Colporrhaphy nec

P24   Repair of vault of vagina
Excludes: Operations to support female bladder (M51-M55)

P24.1   Repair of vault of vagina using combined abdominal and vaginal approach
P24.2   Sacrocolpopexy
P24.3   Repair of vault of vagina using abdominal approach nec
P24.4   Repair of vault of vagina using vaginal approach nec
P24.8   Other specified
P24.9   Unspecified
         Includes: Suspension of vagina nec

P25   Other repair of vagina

P25.1   Repair of vesicovaginal fistula
P25.2   Repair of urethrovaginal fistula
P25.3   Repair of rectovaginal fistula
P25.4   Repair of uterovaginal fistula
P25.5   Suture of vagina
         Includes: Colpoperineorrhaphy
P25.8   Other specified
P25.9   Unspecified

P26   Introduction of supporting pessary into vagina
Excludes: Insertion of abortifacient pessary (Q14.-)

P26.1   Insertion of hodge pessary into vagina
P26.2   Insertion of ring into vagina
P26.3   Removal of supporting pessary from vagina
P26.8   Other specified
P26.9   Unspecified

P27   Exploration of vagina

P27.1   Evacuation of haematoma from vagina
P27.2   Toilet to vagina
P27.3   Colposcopy nec
P27.8   Other specified
P27.9   Unspecified

P29   Other operations on vagina

P29.1   Freeing of adhesions of vagina
P29.2   Colpotomy nec
P29.3   Biopsy of lesion of vagina
         Includes: Biopsy of vagina
P29.4   Removal of foreign body from vagina
P29.5   Dilation of vagina
P29.8   Other specified
P29.9   Unspecified

P31   Operations on pouch of Douglas

P31.1   Culdoplasty
P31.2   Drainage of pouch of Douglas
P31.3   Aspiration of pouch of Douglas
P31.4   Culdotomy nec
P31.5   Removal of intrauterine contraceptive device from pouch of Douglas
P31.6   Removal of foreign body from pouch of Douglas nec
P31.8   Other specified
P31.9   Unspecified

CHAPTER Q

UPPER FEMALE GENITAL TRACT

(CODES Q01-56)

Includes: UTERUS
FALLOPIAN TUBE
OVARY
LIGAMENT OF UTERUS

Excludes: OBSTETRIC OPERATIONS   (Chapter R)
OPERATIONS FOR FEMALE
SEXUAL TRANSFORMATION   (Chapter X)

Note: *Obstetric operations are normally carried out in relation to delivery at or near term or in pregnancy expected to go to term*
They do not include abortion or termination of pregnancy

Q01   **Excision of cervix uteri**

Q01.1   Amputation of cervix uteri
          Excludes: When associated with repair of prolapse of vagina (P22)
Q01.2   Wedge excision of cervix uteri and suture hfq
Q01.3   Excision of lesion of cervix uteri
Q01.8   Other specified
Q01.9   Unspecified

Q02   **Destruction of lesion of cervix uteri**

Q02.1   Avulsion of lesion of cervix uteri
Q02.2   Laser destruction of lesion of cervix uteri
Q02.3   Cauterisation of lesion of cervix uteri
Q02.4   Cryotherapy to lesion of cervix uteri
Q02.8   Other specified
Q02.9   Unspecified

Q03   **Biopsy of cervix uteri**
          Includes: Biopsy of lesion of cervix uteri

Q03.1   Knife cone biopsy of cervix uteri
Q03.2   Laser cone biopsy of cervix uteri
Q03.3   Cone biopsy of cervix uteri nec
Q03.4   Punch biopsy of cervix uteri
Q03.5   Ring biopsy of cervix uteri
Q03.8   Other specified
Q03.9   Unspecified

Q05   **Other operations on cervix uteri**

Q05.1   Repair of cervix uteri nec
          Excludes: Cerclage of cervix of gravid uterus (R12.1)
Q05.2   Dilation of cervix uteri
          Excludes: When associated with curettage of uterus (Q10.1) or other evacuation of uterus (Q11.1 Q11.2)
Q05.8   Other specified
Q05.9   Unspecified

Q07 **Abdominal excision of uterus**
Note: *Use supplementary code for concurrent excision of ovary and/or fallopian tube (Q22-Q24)*

Q07.1 Abdominal hysterocolpectomy and excision of periuterine tissue
Q07.2 Abdominal hysterectomy and excision of periuterine tissue nec
Q07.3 Abdominal hysterocolpectomy nec
Q07.4 Total abdominal hysterectomy nec
    Includes: Hysterectomy nec
Q07.5 Subtotal abdominal hysterectomy
Q07.8 Other specified
Q07.9 Unspecified

Q08 **Vaginal excision of uterus**
Note: *Use as supplementary code when associated with concurrent repair of prolapse of vagina (P23)*
    Use supplementary code for concurrent excision of ovary and/or fallopian tube (Q22-Q24)

Q08.1 Vaginal hysterocolpectomy and excision of periuterine tissue
Q08.2 Vaginal hysterectomy and excision of periuterine tissue nec
Q08.3 Vaginal hysterocolpectomy nec
Q08.8 Other specified
Q08.9 Unspecified
    Includes: Vaginal hysterectomy nec

Q09 **Other open operations on uterus**

Q09.1 Open removal of products of conception from uterus
Q09.2 Open myomectomy
Q09.3 Open excision of lesion of uterus nec
    Includes: Excision of lesion of uterus nec
Q09.4 Open biopsy of lesion of uterus
    Includes: Open biopsy of uterus
Q09.5 Metroplasty
Q09.6 Incision of uterus nec
    Includes: Hysterotomy nec
Q09.8 Other specified
Q09.9 Unspecified

Q10 **Curettage of uterus**

Q10.1 Dilation of cervix uteri and curettage of products of conception from uterus
Q10.2 Curettage of products of conception from uterus nec
Q10.3 Dilation of cervix uteri and curettage of uterus nec
Q10.8 Other specified
Q10.9 Unspecified

Q11 **Other evacuation of contents of uterus**

Q11.1 Dilation of cervix uteri and vacuum aspiration of products of conception from uterus
Q11.2 Dilation of cervix uteri and evacuation of products of conception from uterus nec
Q11.3 Evacuation of products of conception from uterus nec
Q11.4 Extraction of menses
Q11.8 Other specified
Q11.9 Unspecified

Q12 **Intrauterine contraceptive device**

Q12.1 Introduction of intrauterine contraceptive device
Q12.2 Replacement of intrauterine contraceptive device
Q12.3 Removal of displaced intrauterine contraceptive device nec
    Excludes: Removal of displaced intrauterine contraceptive device from pouch of Douglas (P31.5)
Q12.4 Removal of intrauterine contraceptive device nec
Q12.8 Other specified
Q12.9 Unspecified

Q13 **Introduction of gamete into uterine cavity**

Q13.1   Implantation of fertilised egg into uterus
Q13.2   Intracervical artificial insemination
Q13.3   Intrauterine artificial insemination
       Includes: Artificial insemination nec
Q13.8   Other specified
Q13.9   Unspecified

Q14 **Introduction of abortifacient into uterine cavity**

Q14.1   Intraamniotic injection of prostaglandin
Q14.2   Intraamniotic injection of abortifacient nec
Q14.3   Extraamniotic injection of prostaglandin
Q14.4   Extraamniotic injection of abortifacient nec
Q14.5   Insertion of prostaglandin pessary
Q14.6   Insertion of abortifacient pessary nec
Q14.8   Other specified
Q14.9   Unspecified

Q15 **Introduction of other substance into uterine cavity**

Q15.1   Introduction of radioactive substance into uterine cavity
Q15.2   Introduction of therapeutic substance into uterine cavity nec
Q15.3   Injection into uterine cavity nec
Q15.4   Removal of therapeutic substance from uterine cavity
Q15.8   Other specified
Q15.9   Unspecified

Q16 **Other vaginal operations on uterus**

Q16.1   Vaginal excision of lesion of uterus
Q16.8   Other specified
Q16.9   Unspecified

Q17 **Therapeutic endoscopic operations on uterus**
       Note: *It is not necessary to code additionally any mention of diagnostic endoscopic examination of uterus (Q18.9)*

Q17.1   Endoscopic resection of lesion of uterus
Q17.2   Endoscopic cauterisation of lesion of uterus
Q17.3   Endoscopic cryotherapy to lesion of uterus
Q17.4   Endoscopic destruction of lesion of uterus nec
Q17.8   Other specified
Q17.9   Unspecified

Q18 **Diagnostic endoscopic examination of uterus**

Q18.1   Diagnostic endoscopic examination of uterus and biopsy of lesion of uterus
       Includes: Diagnostic endoscopic examination of uterus and biopsy of uterus
                    Endoscopic biopsy of lesion of uterus
                    Endoscopic biopsy of uterus
Q18.8   Other specified
Q18.9   Unspecified
       Includes: Hysteroscopy nec

Q20   Other operations on uterus

Q20.1   Freeing of adhesions of uterus
Q20.2   Biopsy of lesion of uterus nec
         Includes: Biopsy of uterus nec
Q20.3   Manual manipulation of uterus
         Excludes: Manual manipulation of gravid uterus (R12.3) or delivered uterus (R29)
Q20.4   Vaginofixation of uterus
Q20.5   Exploration of uterus nec
Q20.8   Other specified
Q20.9   Unspecified

Q22   Bilateral excision of adnexa of uterus
         Note: Use as supplementary code when associated with concurrent excision of uterus (Q07 Q08)

Q22.1   Bilateral salpingoophorectomy
Q22.2   Bilateral salpingectomy nec
Q22.3   Bilateral oophorectomy nec
Q22.8   Other specified
Q22.9   Unspecified

Q23   Unilateral excision of adnexa of uterus
         Note: Use as supplementary code when associated with concurrent excision of uterus (Q07 Q08)

Q23.1   Unilateral salpingoophorectomy nec
Q23.2   Salpingoophorectomy of remaining solitary fallopian tube and ovary
Q23.3   Unilateral salpingectomy nec
Q23.4   Salpingectomy of remaining solitary fallopian tube nec
Q23.5   Unilateral oophorectomy nec
Q23.6   Oophorectomy of remaining solitary ovary nec
Q23.8   Other specified
Q23.9   Unspecified

Q24   Other excision of adnexa of uterus
         Note: Use as supplementary code when associated with concurrent excision of uterus (Q07 Q08)

Q24.1   Salpingoophorectomy nec
Q24.2   Salpingectomy nec
Q24.3   Oophorectomy nec
Q24.8   Other specified
Q24.9   Unspecified

Q25   Partial excision of fallopian tube
         Excludes: When associated with sterilisation (Q27 Q28)

Q25.1   Excision of lesion of fallopian tube
Q25.8   Other specified
Q25.9   Unspecified
         Includes: Partial salpingectomy nec

Q26   Placement of prosthesis in fallopian tube

Q26.1   Insertion of tubal prosthesis into fallopian tube
Q26.2   Revision of tubal prosthesis in fallopian tube
Q26.3   Removal of tubal prosthesis from fallopian tube
Q26.8   Other specified
Q26.9   Unspecified

Q27   Open bilateral occlusion of fallopian tubes

Q27.1   Open bilateral ligation of fallopian tubes
Q27.2   Open bilateral clipping of fallopian tubes
         Includes: Open bilateral ringing of fallopian tubes
Q27.8   Other specified
Q27.9   Unspecified

Q28 Other open occlusion of fallopian tube

Q28.1 Open ligation of remaining solitary fallopian tube
Q28.2 Open ligation of fallopian tube nec
Q28.3 Open clipping of remaining solitary fallopian tube
Includes: Open ringing of remaining solitary fallopian tube
Q28.4 Open clipping of fallopian tube nec
Includes: Open ringing of fallopian tube nec
Q28.8 Other specified
Q28.9 Unspecified

Q29 Open reversal of female sterilisation

Q29.1 Reanastomosis of fallopian tube nec
Q29.2 Open removal of clip from fallopian tube nec
Includes: Open removal of ring from fallopian tube nec
Q29.8 Other specified
Q29.9 Unspecified

Q30 Other repair of fallopian tube

Q30.1 Reconstruction of fallopian tube
Q30.2 Replantation of fallopian tube
Q30.3 Anastomosis of fallopian tube nec
Q30.4 Salpingostomy
Q30.5 Suture of fallopian tube
Q30.8 Other specified
Q30.9 Unspecified

Q31 Incision of fallopian tube

Q31.1 Removal of products of conception from fallopian tube
Q31.2 Drainage of fallopian tube
Q31.8 Other specified
Q31.9 Unspecified
Includes: Salpingotomy nec

Q32 Operations on fimbria

Q32.1 Excision of fimbria
Q32.2 Burying of fimbria in wall of uterus
Q32.3 Excision of hydatid of Morgagni
Q32.8 Other specified
Q32.9 Unspecified

Q34 Other open operations on fallopian tube

Q34.1 Open freeing of adhesions of fallopian tube
Q34.2 Open biopsy of fallopian tube
Includes: Open biopsy of lesion of fallopian tube
Q34.3 Open dilation of fallopian tube
Q34.4 Exploration of fallopian tube
Q34.8 Other specified
Q34.9 Unspecified

Q35 Endoscopic bilateral occlusion of fallopian tubes
Note: It is not necessary to code additionally any mention of diagnostic endoscopic examination of fallopian tube (Q39.9)

Q35.1 Endoscopic bilateral cauterisation of fallopian tubes
Q35.2 Endoscopic bilateral clipping of fallopian tubes
Q35.3 Endoscopic bilateral ringing of fallopian tubes
Q35.8 Other specified
Q35.9 Unspecified

158

Q36   Other endoscopic occlusion of fallopian tube
         Note: It is not necessary to code additionally any mention of diagnostic endoscopic examination of
                     fallopian tube (Q39.9)

Q36.1   Endoscopic occlusion of remaining solitary fallopian tube
Q36.8   Other specified
Q36.9   Unspecified

Q37   Endoscopic reversal of female sterilisation
         Note: It is not necessary to code additionally any mention of diagnostic endoscopic examination of
                     fallopian tube (Q39.9)

Q37.1   Endoscopic removal of clip from fallopian tube
Q37.8   Other specified
Q37.9   Unspecified

Q38   Other therapeutic endoscopic operations on fallopian tube
         Note: It is not necessary to code additionally any mention of diagnostic endoscopic examination of
                     fallopian tube (Q39.9)

Q38.1   Endoscopic freeing of adhesions of fallopian tube
Q38.2   Endoscopic injection into fallopian tube
Q38.3   Endoscopic intrafallopian transfer of gamete
Q38.8   Other specified
Q38.9   Unspecified

Q39   Diagnostic endoscopic examination of fallopian tube

Q39.1   Diagnostic endoscopic examination of fallopian tube and biopsy of lesion of fallopian tube
         Includes: Diagnostic endoscopic examination of fallopian tube and biopsy of fallopian tube
                   Endoscopic biopsy of lesion of fallopian tube
                   Endoscopic biopsy of fallopian tube
                   Biopsy of lesion of fallopian tube nec
                   Biopsy of fallopian tube nec
Q39.8   Other specified
Q39.9   Unspecified
         Includes: Laparoscopy of fallopian tube nec

Q41   Other operations on fallopian tube

Q41.1   Salpingography
         Includes: Hysterosalpingography
Q41.2   Hydrotubation of fallopian tube
Q41.3   Dye test of fallopian tube
Q41.4   Insufflation of fallopian tube
Q41.5   Operations to ensure patency of fallopian tube nec
         Includes: Dilation of fallopian tube nec
Q41.8   Other specified
Q41.9   Unspecified

Q43   Partial excision of ovary

Q43.1   Excision of wedge of ovary
Q43.2   Excision of lesion of ovary
Q43.3   Marsupialisation of lesion of ovary
Q43.8   Other specified
Q43.9   Unspecified

Q44   Open destruction of lesion of ovary

Q44.1   Open cauterisation of lesion of ovary
Q44.8   Other specified
Q44.9   Unspecified

Q45 Repair of ovary

Q45.1 Replantation of ovary
Q45.2 Fixation of ovary nec
Q45.3 Suture of ovary
Q45.4 Suture of rupture of corpus luteum
Q45.8 Other specified
Q45.9 Unspecified

Q47 Other open operations on ovary

Q47.1 Transposition of ovary
Q47.2 Open freeing of adhesions of ovary
Q47.3 Open biopsy of lesion of ovary
 Includes: Open biopsy of ovary
Q47.4 Open drainage of cyst of ovary
Q47.8 Other specified
Q47.9 Unspecified

Q48 Oocyte recovery

Q48.1 Endoscopic transurethral ultrasound directed oocyte recovery
Q48.2 Endoscopic transvesical oocyte recovery
Q48.3 Laparoscopic oocyte recovery
 Includes: Endoscopic oocyte recovery nec
Q48.4 Transvaginal oocyte recovery
Q48.8 Other specified
Q48.9 Unspecified

Q49 Therapeutic endoscopic operations on ovary
Note: It is not necessary to code additionally any mention of diagnostic endoscopic examination of ovary (Q50.9)

Q49.1 Endoscopic extirpation of lesion of ovary
Q49.2 Endoscopic freeing of adhesions of ovary
Q49.3 Endoscopic drainage of cyst of ovary
Q49.8 Other specified
Q49.9 Unspecified

Q50 Diagnostic endoscopic examination of ovary

Q50.1 Diagnostic endoscopic examination of ovary and biopsy of lesion of ovary
 Includes: Diagnostic endoscopic examination of ovary and biopsy of ovary
  Endoscopic biopsy of lesion of ovary
  Endoscopic biopsy of ovary
  Biopsy of lesion of ovary nec
  Biopsy of ovary nec
Q50.8 Other specified
Q50.9 Unspecified
 Includes: Laparoscopy of ovary nec

Q52 Operations on broad ligament of uterus

Q52.1 Excision of lesion of broad ligament of uterus
Q52.2 Destruction of lesion of broad ligament of uterus
Q52.3 Shortening of broad ligament of uterus
Q52.8 Other specified
Q52.9 Unspecified

Q54 Operations on other ligament of uterus

Q54.1 Suspension of uterus
Q54.2 Plication of round ligament of uterus
Q54.3 Division of uteropelvic ligament
Q54.8 Other specified
Q54.9 Unspecified

Q55   **Other examination of female genital tract**
Includes: Vagina
Cervix uteri
Uterus

Q55.1   Examination of female genital tract under anaesthetic and papanicolau smear
Includes: Examination of female genital tract under anaesthetic and cervical smear
Q55.2   Examination of female genital tract under anaesthetic nec
Q55.3   Papanicolau smear nec
Includes: Cervical smear nec
Q55.8   Other specified
Q55.9   Unspecified
Includes: Gynaecological examination under anaesthetic

Q56   **Other operations on female genital tract**

Q56.1   Fertility investigation of female nec
Excludes: Patency operations on fallopian tube (Q41)
Q56.8   Other specified
Q56.9   Unspecified

161

CHAPTER R

FEMALE GENITAL TRACT ASSOCIATED
WITH PREGNANCY CHILDBIRTH AND PUERPERIUM

(CODES R01-R34)

Excludes: OPERATIONS ASSOCIATED WITH
          PREGNANCY WITH ABORTIVE OUTCOME   (Chapter Q)

R01   **Therapeutic endoscopic operations on fetus**
        Note: *It is not necessary to code additionally any mention of diagnostic endoscopic examination of fetus (R02.9)*

R01.1   Fetoscopic blood transfusion of fetus
R01.8   Other specified
R01.9   Unspecified

R02   **Diagnostic endoscopic examination of fetus**

R02.1   Fetoscopic examination of fetus and fetoscopic biopsy of fetus
        Includes: Fetoscopic biopsy of fetus nec
R02.2   Fetoscopic examination of fetus and fetoscopic sampling of fetal blood
        Includes: Fetoscopic sampling of fetal blood nec
R02.8   Other specified
R02.9   Unspecified
        Includes: Fetoscopy nec

R03   **Selective destruction of fetus**
        Note: *Use subsidiary code to identify method of image control as necessary (Y53)*

R03.1   Early selective feticide
R03.2   Late selective feticide
R03.8   Other specified
R03.9   Unspecified
        Includes: Selective feticide nec

R04   **Therapeutic percutaneous operations on fetus**
        Note: *Use subsidiary code to identify method of image control as necessary (Y53)*

R04.1   Percutaneous insertion of fetal vesicoamniotic shunt
R04.2   Percutaneous insertion of fetal pleuroamniotic shunt
R04.3   Percutaneous blood transfusion of fetus
R04.8   Other specified
R04.9   Unspecified

R05   **Diagnostic percutaneous examination of fetus**
        Includes: .Placenta
        Note: *Use subsidiary code to identify method of image control as necessary (Y53)*

R05.1   Percutaneous biopsy of fetus
R05.2   Percutaneous sampling of fetal blood
R05.3   Percutaneous sampling of chorionic villus
R05.8   Other specified
R05.9   Unspecified

R10   **Other operations on amniotic cavity**
        Note: *Use subsidiary code to identify method of image control as necessary (Y53)*

R10.1   Drainage of amniotic cavity
R10.2   Diagnostic amniocentesis
        Includes: Amniocentesis nec
R10.3   Amnioscopy
R10.4   Sampling of chorionic villus nec
        Includes: Sampling of chorionic villus using vaginal approach
R10.5   Biopsy of placenta nec
R10.8   Other specified
R10.9   Unspecified

R12   **Operations on gravid uterus**

R12.1   Cerclage of cervix of gravid uterus
R12.2   Removal of cerclage from cervix of gravid uterus
R12.3   Repositioning of retroverted gravid uterus
R12.8   Other specified
R12.9   Unspecified

R14   **Surgical induction of labour**

R14.1   Fore water rupture of amniotic membrane
R14.2   Hind water rupture of amniotic membrane
R14.8   Other specified
R14.9   Unspecified

R15   **Other induction of labour**

R15.1   Oxytocic induction of labour
        Includes: Induction of labour using prostaglandins
R15.8   Other specified
R15.9   Unspecified

R17   **Elective caesarean delivery**

R17.1   Elective upper uterine segment caesarean delivery
R17.2   Elective lower uterine segment caesarean delivery
R17.8   Other specified
R17.9   Unspecified

R18   **Other caesarean delivery**
        Excludes: Caesarean hysterectomy (R25.1)

R18.1   Upper uterine segment caesarean delivery nec
R18.2   Lower uterine segment caesarean delivery nec
R18.8   Other specified
R18.9   Unspecified

R19   **Breech extraction delivery**

R19.1   Breech extraction delivery with version
R19.8   Other specified
R19.9   Unspecified

R20   **Other breech delivery**

R20.1   Spontaneous breech delivery
R20.2   Assisted breech delivery
R20.8   Other specified
R20.9   Unspecified

R21 **Forceps cephalic delivery**

R21.1 High forceps cephalic delivery with rotation
R21.2 High forceps cephalic delivery nec
R21.3 Mid forceps cephalic delivery with rotation
R21.4 Mid forceps cephalic delivery nec
R21.5 Low forceps cephalic delivery
R21.8 Other specified
R21.9 Unspecified

R22 **Vacuum delivery**

R22.1 High vacuum delivery
R22.2 Low vacuum delivery
R22.3 Vacuum delivery before full dilation of cervix
R22.8 Other specified
R22.9 Unspecified

R23 **Cephalic vaginal delivery with abnormal presentation of head at delivery without instrument**

R23.1 Manipulative cephalic vaginal delivery with abnormal presentation of head at delivery without instrument
R23.2 Non manipulative cephalic vaginal delivery with abnormal presentation of head at delivery without instrument
R23.8 Other specified
R23.9 Unspecified

R24 **Normal delivery**

R24.9 All

R25 **Other methods of delivery**

R25.1 Caesarean hysterectomy
R25.2 Destructive operation to facilitate delivery
R25.8 Other specified
R25.9 Unspecified

R27 **Other operations to facilitate delivery**

R27.1 Episiotomy to facilitate delivery
R27.8 Other specified
R27.9 Unspecified

R28 **Instrumental removal of products of conception from delivered uterus**
Excludes: After termination of pregnancy (Q10 Q11)

R28.1 Curettage of delivered uterus
R28.8 Other specified
R28.9 Unspecified

R29 **Manual removal of products of conception from delivered uterus**
Excludes: Expression of placenta (R30.2)

R29.1 Manual removal of placenta from delivered uterus
R29.8 Other specified
R29.9 Unspecified

R30 **Other operations on delivered uterus**

R30.1 Repositioning of inverted delivered uterus
R30.2 Expression of placenta
R30.3 Instrumental exploration of delivered uterus nec
R30.4 Manual exploration of delivered uterus nec
       Includes: Exploration of delivered uterus nec
R30.8 Other specified
R30.9 Unspecified

R32   Immediate repair of obstetric laceration

R32.1   Immediate repair of obstetric laceration of uterus or cervix uteri
R32.2   Immediate repair of obstetric laceration of perineum and sphincter of anus
R32.3   Immediate repair of obstetric laceration of vagina and floor of pelvis
R32.4   Immediate repair of minor obstetric laceration
R32.8   Other specified
R32.9   Unspecified

R34   Other obstetric operations

R34.8   Other specified
R34.9   Unspecified

CHAPTERS

SKIN

(CODES S01-S70)

Note: **Codes from this chapter are not to be used as primary codes for following skin sites:**

SKIN SITE	CHAPTER	CODE
NIPPLE	B	B35
EYEBROW	C	C10
LIP	F	F01-F06

and for skin of following sites:

SITE	CHAPTER	CODE
EYELID	C	C12 C17 C19 C22
EXTERNAL EAR	D	D01-D06
EXTERNAL NOSE	E	E09
SCROTUM	N	N01-N03
MALE PERINEUM	N	N24
PENIS	N	N27-N28 N32
Includes: Prepuce	N	N30
VULVA	P	P05-P09
FEMALE PERINEUM	P	P11-P13
UMBILICUS	T	T29

Codes from this chapter may however be used to enhance these codes where necessary

S01   **Plastic excision of skin of head or neck**
Includes: Subcutaneous tissue of head or neck

S01.1   Facelift and tightening of platysma
S01.2   Facelift nec
S01.3   Submental lipectomy
S01.4   Browlift
S01.8   Other specified
S01.9   Unspecified

S02   **Plastic excision of skin of abdominal wall**
Includes: Subcutaneous tissue of abdominal wall
Excludes: Plastic excision of skin of umbilicus (T29.6)

S02.1   Abdominoplasty
S02.2   Abdominolipectomy
S02.8   Other specified
S02.9   Unspecified

S03   **Plastic excision of skin of other site**
Includes: Subcutaneous tissue nec

S03.1   Buttock lift
S03.2   Thigh lift
S03.3   Excision of redundant skin or fat of arm
S03.8   Other specified
S03.9   Unspecified

S04   Other excision of skin

S04.1   Excision of sweat gland bearing skin of axilla
S04.2   Excision of sweat gland bearing skin of groin
S04.3   Excision of sweat gland bearing skin nec
           Excludes: Excision of sweat gland bearing skin of male perineum (N24.1) or female perineum (P13.7)
S04.8   Other specified
S04.9   Unspecified

S05   Microscopically controlled excision of lesion of skin
           Includes: Subcutaneous tissue

S05.1   Microscopically controlled excision of lesion of skin of head or neck using fresh tissue technique
S05.2   Microscopically controlled excision of lesion of skin using fresh tissue technique nec
S05.3   Microscopically controlled excision of lesion of skin of head or neck using chemosurgical technique
S05.4   Microscopically controlled excision of lesion of skin using chemosurgical technique nec
S05.5   Microscopically controlled excision of lesion of skin of head or neck nec
S05.8   Other specified
S05.9   Unspecified

S06   Other excision of lesion of skin
           Includes: Subcutaneous tissue

S06.1   Marsupialisation of lesion of skin of head or neck
S06.2   Marsupialisation of lesion of skin nec
S06.3   Shave excision of lesion of skin of head or neck
S06.4   Shave excision of lesion of skin nec
S06.5   Excision of lesion of skin of head or neck nec
S06.8   Other specified
S06.9   Unspecified

S08   Curettage of lesion of skin
           Includes: Subcutaneous tissue

S08.1   Curettage and cauterisation of lesion of skin of head or neck
S08.2   Curettage and cauterisation of lesion of skin nec
S08.3   Curettage of lesion of skin of head or neck nec
S08.8   Other specified
S08.9   Unspecified

S09   Photodestruction of lesion of skin
           Includes: Subcutaneous tissue

S09.1   Laser destruction of lesion of skin of head or neck
S09.2   Laser destruction of lesion of skin nec
S09.3   Photodestruction of lesion of skin of head or neck nec
S09.8   Other specified
S09.9   Unspecified

S10   Other destruction of lesion of skin of head or neck
           Includes: Subcutaneous tissue

S10.1   Cauterisation of lesion of skin of head or neck nec
S10.2   Cryotherapy to lesion of skin of head or neck
S10.3   Chemical peeling of lesion of skin of head or neck
S10.4   Electrolysis to lesion of skin of head or neck
S10.8   Other specified
S10.9   Unspecified

S11 **Other destruction of lesion of skin of other site**
Includes: Subcutaneous tissue

S11.1 Cauterisation of lesion of skin nec
S11.2 Cryotherapy to lesion of skin nec
S11.3 Chemical peeling of lesion of skin nec
S11.4 Electrolysis to lesion of skin nec
S11.8 Other specified
S11.9 Unspecified

S13 **Punch biopsy of skin**

S13.1 Punch biopsy of lesion of skin of head or neck
S13.2 Punch biopsy of lesion of skin nec
S13.8 Other specified
S13.9 Unspecified

S14 **Shave biopsy of skin**

S14.1 Shave biopsy of lesion of skin of head or neck
S14.2 Shave biopsy of lesion of skin nec
S14.8 Other specified
S14.9 Unspecified

S15 **Other biopsy of skin**
Includes: Subcutaneous tissue

S15.1 Biopsy of lesion of skin of head or neck nec
S15.2 Biopsy of lesion of skin nec
S15.8 Other specified
S15.9 Unspecified

S17 **Distant flap of skin and muscle**

S17.1 Distant myocutaneous subcutaneous pedicle flap to head or neck
S17.2 Distant myocutaneous subcutaneous pedicle flap nec
S17.3 Distant myocutaneous flap to head or neck nec
S17.8 Other specified
S17.9 Unspecified
       Includes: Distant myocutaneous flap nec

S18 **Distant flap of skin and fascia**

S18.1 Distant fasciocutaneous subcutaneous pedicle flap to head or neck
S18.2 Distant fasciocutaneous subcutaneous pedicle flap nec
S18.3 Distant fasciocutaneous flap to head or neck nec
S18.8 Other specified
S18.9 Unspecified
       Includes: Distant fasciocutaneous flap nec

S19 **Distant pedicle flap of skin**

S19.1 Distant tube pedicle flap of skin to head or neck
S19.2 Distant tube pedicle flap of skin nec
S19.8 Other specified
S19.9 Unspecified

S20 **Other distant flap of skin**

S20.1 Axial pattern distant flap of skin to head or neck
S20.2 Axial pattern distant flap of skin nec
S20.3 Random pattern distant flap of skin to head or neck
S20.4 Random pattern distant flap of skin nec
S20.5 Distant flap of skin to head or neck nec
S20.8 Other specified
S20.9 Unspecified

S21   **Hair bearing flap of skin**
Excludes: Hair bearing flap of skin to eyebrow (C10.2)

S21.1   Hair bearing flap of skin to scalp for male pattern baldness
S21.2   Hair bearing flap of skin to scalp nec
S21.3   Hair bearing flap of skin to nasolabial area
S21.4   Hair bearing flap of skin to chin area
S21.8   Other specified
S21.9   Unspecified

S22   **Sensory flap of skin**

S22.1   Neurovascular island sensory flap of skin to head or neck
S22.2   Neurovascular island sensory flap of skin nec
S22.3   Local sensory flap of skin to head or neck
S22.4   Local sensory flap of skin nec
S22.8   Other specified
S22.9   Unspecified

S23   **Flap operations to relax contracture of skin**

S23.1   Z plasty to head or neck
S23.2   Z plasty nec
S23.3   W plasty to head or neck
S23.4   W plasty nec
S23.8   Other specified
S23.9   Unspecified

S24   **Local flap of skin and muscle**
Includes: Myocutaneous flap nec

S24.1   Local myocutaneous subcutaneous pedicle flap to head or neck
S24.2   Local myocutaneous subcutaneous pedicle flap nec
S24.3   Local myocutaneous flap to head or neck nec
S24.8   Other specified
S24.9   Unspecified
Includes: Local myocutaneous flap nec

S25   **Local flap of skin and fascia**
Includes: Fasciocutaneous flap nec

S25.1   Local fasciocutaneous subcutaneous pedicle flap to head or neck
S25.2   Local fasciocutaneous subcutaneous pedicle flap nec
S25.3   Local fasciocutaneous flap to head or neck nec
S25.8   Other specified
S25.9   Unspecified
Includes: Local fasciocutaneous flap nec

S26   **Local subcutaneous pedicle flap of skin**
Includes: Subcutaneous pedicle flap of skin nec

S26.1   Axial pattern local subcutaneous pedicle flap of skin to head or neck
S26.2   Axial pattern local subcutaneous pedicle flap of skin nec
S26.3   Random pattern local subcutaneous pedicle flap of skin to head or neck
S26.4   Random pattern local subcutaneous pedicle flap of skin nec
S26.5   Local subcutaneous pedicle flap of skin to head or neck nec
S26.8   Other specified
S26.9   Unspecified

S27   **Other local flap of skin**
         Includes: Flap of skin nec

S27.1   Axial pattern local flap of skin to head or neck nec
S27.2   Axial pattern local flap of skin nec
S27.3   Random pattern local flap of skin to head or neck nec
S27.4   Random pattern local flap of skin nec
S27.5   Local flap of skin to head or neck nec
S27.8   Other specified
S27.9   Unspecified

S28   **Flap of mucosa**

S28.1   Tongue flap
S28.8   Other specified
S28.9   Unspecified

S30   **Other operations on flap of skin to head or neck**

S30.1   Delay of flap of skin to head or neck
S30.2   Transfer of flap of skin to head or neck
S30.3   Revision of flap of skin to head or neck
S30.4   Final inset of flap of skin to head or neck
S30.5   Thinning of flap of skin to head or neck
S30.6   Removal of flap of skin to head or neck
S30.8   Other specified
S30.9   Unspecified

S31   **Other operations on flap of skin to other site**

S31.1   Delay of flap of skin nec
S31.2   Transfer of flap of skin nec
S31.3   Revision of flap of skin nec
S31.4   Final inset of flap of skin nec
S31.5   Thinning of flap of skin nec
S31.6   Removal of flap of skin nec
S31.8   Other specified
S31.9   Unspecified

S33   **Hair bearing graft of skin to scalp**

S33.1   Hair bearing punch graft to scalp for male pattern baldness
S33.2   Hair bearing strip graft to scalp for male pattern baldness
S33.3   Hair bearing graft to scalp for male pattern baldness nec
S33.8   Other specified
S33.9   Unspecified

S34   **Hair bearing graft of skin to other site**
         Excludes: Hair bearing graft to eyebrow (C10.3)

S34.1   Hair bearing graft to nasolabial area
S34.2   Hair bearing graft to chin area
S34.8   Other specified
S34.9   Unspecified

S35   **Split autograft of skin**

S35.1   Meshed split autograft of skin to head or neck
S35.2   Meshed split autograft of skin nec
S35.3   Split autograft of skin to head or neck nec
S35.8   Other specified
S35.9   Unspecified

S36   **Other autograft of skin**

S36.1   Full thickness autograft of skin to head or neck
S36.2   Full thickness autograft of skin nec
S36.3   Composite autograft of skin to head or neck
S36.4   Composite autograft of skin nec
S36.5   Pinch graft of skin to head or neck
S36.6   Pinch graft of skin nec
S36.8   Other specified
S36.9   Unspecified

S37   **Other graft of skin**

S37.1   Allograft of skin to head or neck
S37.2   Allograft of skin nec
S37.3   Xenograft of skin to head or neck
S37.4   Xenograft of skin nec
S37.8   Other specified
S37.9   Unspecified

S38   **Graft of mucosa**

S38.1   Graft of mucosa to head or neck
S38.8   Other specified
S38.9   Unspecified

S39   **Graft of other tissue to skin**
           Includes: Graft of tissue to subcutaneous tissue

S39.1   Allograft of amniotic membrane to head or neck
S39.2   Allograft of amniotic membrane nec
S39.8   Other specified
S39.9   Unspecified

S41   **Suture of skin of head or neck**
           Includes: Insertion of clip into skin of head or neck
           Subcutaneous tissue of head or neck
           Wound of head or neck

S41.1   Primary suture of skin of head or neck nec
S41.2   Delayed primary suture of skin of head or neck
S41.3   Secondary suture of skin of head or neck
S41.4   Resuture of skin of head or neck
S41.8   Other specified
S41.9   Unspecified

S42   **Suture of skin of other site**
           Includes: Insertion of clip into skin nec
           Subcutaneous tissue nec
           Wound nec

S42.1   Primary suture of skin nec
S42.2   Delayed primary suture of skin nec
S42.3   Secondary suture of skin nec
S42.4   Resuture of skin nec
S42.8   Other specified
S42.9   Unspecified

S43   **Removal of repair material from skin**
Includes: Subcutaneous tissue
Wound

S43.1   Removal of clip from skin of head or neck
S43.2   Removal of clip from skin nec
S43.3   Removal of suture from skin of head or neck
S43.4   Removal of suture from skin nec
S43.8   Other specified
S43.9   Unspecified

S44   **Removal of other inorganic substance from skin**
Includes: Subcutaneous tissue
Wound

S44.1   Removal of metal from skin of head or neck
S44.2   Removal of metal from skin nec
S44.3   Removal of glass from skin of head or neck
S44.4   Removal of glass from skin nec
S44.5   Removal of inorganic foreign body from skin of head or neck nec
S44.6   Removal of inorganic foreign body from skin nec
S44.8   Other specified
S44.9   Unspecified

S45   **Removal of other substance from skin**
Includes: Subcutaneous tissue
Wound

S45.1   Removal of dirt from skin of head or neck
S45.2   Removal of dirt from skin nec
S45.3   Removal of organic material from skin of head or neck nec
S45.4   Removal of organic material from skin nec
S45.5   Removal of foreign body from skin of head or neck nec
S45.6   Removal of foreign body from skin nec
S45.8   Other specified
S45.9   Unspecified

S47   **Opening of skin**
Includes: Subcutaneous tissue

S47.1   Drainage of lesion of skin of head or neck
S47.2   Drainage of lesion of skin nec
S47.3   Incision of lesion of skin of head or neck
S47.4   Incision of lesion of skin nec
S47.5   Incision of skin of head or neck
S47.6   Incision of skin nec
S47.8   Other specified
S47.9   Unspecified

S48   **Insertion of skin expander into subcutaneous tissue**

S48.1   Insertion of skin expander into subcutaneous tissue of head or neck
S48.2   Insertion of skin expander into subcutaneous tissue of breast
S48.8   Other specified
S48.9   Unspecified

S49   **Attention to skin expander in subcutaneous tissue**

S49.1   Adjustment to skin expander in subcutaneous tissue
S49.2   Removal of skin expander from subcutaneous tissue of head or neck
S49.3   Removal of skin expander from subcutaneous tissue of breast
S49.4   Removal of skin expander from subcutaneous tissue nec
S49.8   Other specified
S49.9   Unspecified

S50   **Introduction of other inert substance into subcutaneous tissue**

S50.1   Insertion of organic inert substance into subcutaneous tissue
S50.2   Injection of organic inert substance into subcutaneous tissue
S50.3   Insertion of inert substance into subcutaneous tissue nec
S50.4   Injection of inert substance into subcutaneous tissue nec
S50.8   Other specified
S50.9   Unspecified

S51   **Introduction of destructive substance into subcutaneous tissue**

S51.1   Injection of sclerosing substance into subcutaneous tissue
S51.8   Other specified
S51.9   Unspecified

S52   **Introduction of therapeutic substance into subcutaneous tissue**

S52.1   Insertion of steroid into subcutaneous tissue
S52.2   Injection of steroid into subcutaneous tissue
S52.3   Insertion of therapeutic substance into subcutaneous tissue nec
S52.4   Injection of therapeutic substance into subcutaneous tissue nec
S52.8   Other specified
S52.9   Unspecified

S53   **Introduction of substance into skin**

S53.1   Insertion of therapeutic substance into skin
S53.2   Injection of therapeutic substance into skin
S53.3   Insertion of inert substance into skin
S53.4   Injection of inert substance into skin
S53.8   Other specified
S53.9   Unspecified

S54   **Exploration of burnt skin of head or neck**
         Includes: Subcutaneous tissue of head or neck

S54.1   Debridement of burnt skin of head or neck
S54.2   Removal of slough from burnt skin of head or neck
         Includes: Escharotomy of burnt skin of head or neck
S54.3   Toilet to burnt skin of head or neck nec
S54.4   Dressing of burnt skin of head or neck
S54.5   Attention to dressing of burnt skin of head or neck
S54.8   Other specified
S54.9   Unspecified

S55   **Exploration of burnt skin of other site**
         Includes: Subcutaneous tissue nec

S55.1   Debridement of burnt skin nec
S55.2   Removal of slough from burnt skin nec
         Includes: Escharotomy of burnt skin nec
S55.3   Toilet to burnt skin nec
S55.4   Dressing of burnt skin nec
S55.5   Attention to dressing of burnt skin nec
S55.8   Other specified
S55.9   Unspecified

S56   **Exploration of other skin of head or neck**
Includes: Subcutaneous tissue of head or neck nec
Wound of head or neck nec

S56.1   Debridement of skin of head or neck nec
Includes: Excision of devitalised skin of head or neck nec
S56.2   Removal of slough from skin of head or neck nec
Includes: Escharotomy of skin of head or neck nec
S56.3   Toilet to skin of head or neck nec
S56.4   Dressing of skin of head or neck nec
S56.5   Attention to dressing of skin of head or neck nec
S56.8   Other specified
S56.9   Unspecified

S57   **Exploration of other skin of other site**
Includes: Subcutaneous tissue nec
Wound nec

S57.1   Debridement of skin nec
Includes: Excision of devitalised skin nec
S57.2   Removal of slough from skin nec
Includes: Escharotomy of skin nec
S57.3   Toilet of skin nec
S57.4   Dressing of skin nec
S57.5   Attention to dressing of skin nec
S57.8   Other specified
S57.9   Unspecified

S60   **Other operations on skin**
Includes: Wound

S60.1   Dermabrasion of skin of head or neck
S60.2   Dermabrasion of skin nec
S60.3   Tattooing of skin
S60.4   Refashioning of scar nec
S60.8   Other specified
S60.9   Unspecified

S62   **Other operations on subcutaneous tissue**

S62.1   Liposuction of subcutaneous tissue of head or neck
S62.2   Liposuction of subcutaneous tissue nec
S62.3   Removal of inserted substance from subcutaneous tissue
S62.4   Removal of pack from subcutaneous tissue
S62.8   Other specified
S62.9   Unspecified

S64   **Extirpation of nail bed**

S64.1   Excision of nail bed
S64.2   Chemical destruction of nail bed
S64.3   Destruction of nail bed nec
S64.8   Other specified
S64.9   Unspecified

S66   **Other operations on nail bed**

S66.1   Biopsy of lesion of nail bed
Includes: Biopsy of nail bed
S66.2   Repair of nail bed
S66.3   Incision of nail bed
S66.8   Other specified
S66.9   Unspecified

S68   Excision of nail

S68.1   Total excision of nail
S68.2   Excision of wedge of nail
S68.3   Partial excision of nail nec
S68.8   Other specified
S68.9   Unspecified

S70   Other operations on nail

S70.1   Avulsion of nail
         Includes: Removal of nail nec
S70.2   Incision of nail
S70.3   Removal of foreign body from nail
S70.8   Other specified
S70.9   Unspecified

CHAPTER T

SOFT TISSUE

(CODES T01-T96)

Includes: CHEST WALL
ABDOMINAL WALL
FASCIA
TENDON
MUSCLE
LYMPHATIC TISSUE
CONNECTIVE TISSUE

Excludes: MUSCLE OF EYE   (Chapter C)
SOME OPERATIONS ON SOFT TISSUE FOR CORRECTION
OF CONGENITAL DEFORMITY OF LIMB   (Chapter X)

T01   Partial excision of chest wall

T01.1   Thoracoplasty
T01.2   Removal of plombage material from chest wall
T01.3   Excision of lesion of chest wall
T01.8   Other specified
T01.9   Unspecified

T02   Reconstruction of chest wall

T02.1   Correction of pectus deformity of chest wall
        Includes: Correction of pectus carinatum
        Correction of pectus excavatum
T02.2   Insertion of silicone implant for correction of pectus excavatum
T02.3   Insertion of prosthesis into chest wall nec
T02.4   Removal of prosthesis from chest wall
T02.8   Other specified
T02.9   Unspecified

T03   Opening of chest
        Includes: Chest wall
        Pleura
        Pleural cavity
        Note: Do not use as approach code (Y49)

T03.1   Exploratory median sternotomy
T03.2   Reopening of chest and reexploration of intraabdominal operation site and surgical arrest of postoperative
        bleeding
        Includes: Reopening of incision of chest and reexploration of intraabdominal operation site and surgical
        arrest of bleeding
        Reopening of wound of chest and reexploration of intraabdominal operation site and surgical
        arrest of bleeding
T03.3   Reopening of chest and reexploration of intraabdominal operation site nec
        Includes: Reopening of incision of chest and reexploration of intraabdominal operation site nec
        Reopening of wound of chest and reexploration of intraabdominal operation site nec
T03.4   Reopening of chest nec
        Includes: Reopening of incision of chest nec
        Reopening of wound of chest nec
T03.8   Other specified
T03.9   Unspecified
        Includes: Exploratory thoracotomy nec

T05 **Other operations on chest wall**

T05.1   Suture of chest wall
T05.2   Resuture of previous incision of chest wall
        Includes: Resuture of rupture of incision of chest wall
        Suture of dehiscence of wound of chest wall
T05.3   Repair of chest wall nec
T05.4   Removal of wire from chest wall
T05.8   Other specified
T05.9   Unspecified

T07 **Open excision of pleura**

T07.1   Decortication of pleura
T07.2   Open excision of lesion of pleura
T07.8   Other specified
T07.9   Unspecified
        Includes: Pleurectomy nec

T08 **Open drainage of pleural cavity**

T08.1   Resection of rib and open drainage of pleural cavity
T08.2   Closure of open drainage of pleural cavity
T08.3   Fenestration of pleura
T08.4   Closure of fenestration of pleura
T08.8   Other specified
T08.9   Unspecified

T09 **Other open operations on pleura**

T09.1   Open destruction of lesion of pleura
T09.2   Open biopsy of lesion of pleura
        Includes: Open biopsy of pleura
T09.3   Mechanical open pleurodesis
T09.4   Chemical open pleurodesis
T09.5   Open pleurodesis nec
T09.8   Other specified
T09.9   Unspecified

T10 **Therapeutic endoscopic operations on pleura**
        Note: *It is not necessary to code additionally any mention of diagnostic endoscopic examination of pleural cavity (T11.9)*
        Therapeutic endoscopic operations specifically directed at individual intrathoracic organs are usually classified elsewhere

T10.1   Endoscopic extirpation of lesion of pleura
T10.2   Endoscopic pleurodesis using talc
T10.3   Endoscopic pleurodesis nec
T10.8   Other specified
T10.9   Unspecified

T11 **Diagnostic endoscopic examination of pleura**
        Includes: Pleural cavity
        Note: *Diagnostic endoscopic examinations specifically directed at individual intrathoracic organs are usually classified elsewhere*

T11.1   Diagnostic endoscopic examination of pleura and biopsy of lesion of pleura
        Includes: Diagnostic endoscopic examination of pleura and biopsy of pleura
        Endoscopic biopsy of lesion of pleura
        Endoscopic biopsy of pleura
T11.2   Diagnostic endoscopic examination of pleura and biopsy of lesion of intrathoracic organ nec
        Includes: Diagnostic endoscopic examination of pleura and biopsy of intrathoracic organ nec
        Thoracoscopic biopsy of lesion of intrathoracic organ nec
        Thoracoscopic biopsy of intrathoracic organ nec
        Note: *Use subsidiary site code as necessary*
T11.8   Other specified
T11.9   Unspecified
        Includes: Thoracoscopy nec

T12   **Puncture of pleura**

T12.1   Drainage of lesion of pleura nec
        Includes: Drainage of lesion of pleural cavity nec
T12.2   Drainage of pleural cavity nec
        Includes: Paracentesis of chest
        Excludes: Insertion of underwater drain into chest (T12.4)
T12.3   Aspiration of pleural cavity
        Includes: Thoracocentesis
T12.4   Insertion of tube drain into pleural cavity
        Includes: Insertion of underwater drain into chest
T12.8   Other specified
T12.9   Unspecified

T13   **Introduction of substance into pleural cavity**

T13.1   Insufflation of talc into pleural cavity nec
T13.2   Introduction of sclerosing substance into pleural cavity nec
T13.3   Introduction of cytotoxic substance into pleural cavity
T13.4   Introduction of therapeutic substance into pleural cavity
T13.8   Other specified
T13.9   Unspecified

T14   **Other operations on pleura**
        Includes: Pleural cavity

T14.1   Percutaneous biopsy of lesion of pleura
        Includes: Percutaneous biopsy of pleura
        Biopsy of lesion of pleura nec
        Biopsy of pleura nec
T14.8   Other specified
T14.9   Unspecified

T15   **Repair of rupture of diaphragm**

T15.1   Repair of traumatic rupture of diaphragm
T15.2   Repair of postoperative rupture of diaphragm
T15.8   Other specified
T15.9   Unspecified

T16   **Other repair of diaphragm**
        Excludes: Repair of hiatus hernia (G23)

T16.1   Insertion of prosthesis for repair of diaphragm
T16.2   Plication of diaphragm
T16.3   Closure of fistula of diaphragm
T16.4   Repair of congenital diaphragmatic hernia
T16.5   Suture of diaphragm nec
T16.8   Other specified
T16.9   Unspecified

T17   **Other operations on diaphragm**

T17.1   Excision of lesion of diaphragm
T17.2   Destruction of lesion of diaphragm
T17.8   Other specified
T17.9   Unspecified

T19 Simple excision of inguinal hernial sac
    Note: Use supplementary code as necessary for tether of testis (N13.2)

T19.1   Bilateral herniotomy
T19.2   Unilateral herniotomy
T19.3   Ligation of patent processus vaginalis
    Includes: Correction of hydrocele of infancy
T19.8   Other specified
T19.9   Unspecified
    Includes: Herniotomy nec

T20 Primary repair of inguinal hernia
    Includes: Repair of inguinal hernia nec
    Note: Use supplementary code as necessary for concurrent excision of bowel (eg G69.3 H11.1)
    Use supplementary code as necessary for relief of strangulation of bowel (eg G76.2 H17.5)
    Use subsidiary code to identify primary bilateral repair of inguinal herniae (Z94)

T20.1   Primary repair of inguinal hernia using insert of natural material
T20.2   Primary repair of inguinal hernia using insert of prosthetic material
    Includes: Primary repair of inguinal hernia using insert nec
T20.3   Primary repair of inguinal hernia using sutures
T20.4   Primary repair of inguinal hernia and reduction of sliding hernia
T20.8   Other specified
T20.9   Unspecified

T21 Repair of recurrent inguinal hernia
    Note: Use supplementary code as necessary for concurrent excision of bowel (eg G69.3 H11.1)
    Use supplementary code as necessary for relief of strangulation of bowel (eg G76.2 H17.5)
    Use subsidiary code to identify bilateral repair of recurrent inguinal herniae (Z94)

T21.1   Repair of recurrent inguinal hernia using insert of natural material
T21.2   Repair of recurrent inguinal hernia using insert of prosthetic material
    Includes: Repair of recurrent inguinal hernia using insert nec
T21.3   Repair of recurrent inguinal hernia using sutures
T21.4   Removal of prosthetic material from previous repair of inguinal hernia
T21.8   Other specified
T21.9   Unspecified

T22 Primary repair of femoral hernia
    Includes: Repair of femoral hernia nec
    Note: Use supplementary code as necessary for concurrent excision of bowel (eg G69.3 H11.1)
    Use supplementary code as necessary for relief of strangulation of bowel (eg G76.2 H17.5)
    Use subsidiary code to identify bilateral repair of femoral herniae (Z94)

T22.1   Primary repair of femoral hernia using insert of natural material
T22.2   Primary repair of femoral hernia using insert of prosthetic material
    Includes: Primary repair of femoral hernia using insert nec
T22.3   Primary repair of femoral hernia using sutures
T22.8   Other specified
T22.9   Unspecified

T23 Repair of recurrent femoral hernia
    Note: Use supplementary code as necessary for concurrent excision of bowel (eg G69.3 H11.1)
    Use supplementary code as necessary for relief of strangulation of bowel (eg G76.2 H17.5)
    Use subsidiary code to identify bilateral repair of recurrent femoral herniae (Z94)

T23.1   Repair of recurrent femoral hernia using insert of natural material
T23.2   Repair of recurrent femoral hernia using insert of prosthetic material
    Includes: Repair of recurrent femoral hernia using insert nec
T23.3   Repair of recurrent femoral hernia using sutures
T23.4   Removal of prosthetic material from previous repair of femoral hernia
T23.8   Other specified
T23.9   Unspecified

T24   **Repair of umbilical hernia**

T24.1   Repair of umbilical hernia using insert of natural material
T24.2   Repair of umbilical hernia using insert of prosthetic material
         Includes: Repair of umbilical hernia using insert nec
T24.3   Repair of umbilical hernia using sutures
T24.4   Removal of prosthetic material from previous repair of umbilical hernia
T24.8   Other specified
T24.9   Unspecified

T25   **Primary repair of incisional hernia**
         Includes: Repair of incisional hernia nec
         Note: Use supplementary code as necessary for concurrent excision of bowel (eg G69.3 H11.1)
         *   Use supplementary code as necessary for relief of strangulation of bowel (eg G76.2 H17.5)*

T25.1   Primary repair of incisional hernia using insert of natural material
T25.2   Primary repair of incisional hernia using insert of prosthetic material
         Includes: Primary repair of incisional hernia using insert nec
T25.3   Primary repair of incisional hernia using sutures
T25.8   Other specified
T25.9   Unspecified

T26   **Repair of recurrent incisional hernia**
         Note: Use supplementary code as necessary for concurrent excision of bowel (eg G69.3 H11.1)
         *   Use supplementary code as necessary for relief of strangulation of bowel (eg G76.2 H17.5)*

T26.1   Repair of recurrent incisional hernia using insert of natural material
T26.2   Repair of recurrent incisional hernia using insert of prosthetic material
         Includes: Repair of recurrent incisional hernia using insert nec
T26.3   Repair of recurrent incisional hernia using sutures
T26.4   Removal of prosthetic material from previous repair of incisional hernia
T26.8   Other specified
T26.9   Unspecified

T27   **Repair of other hernia of abdominal wall**
         Note: Use supplementary code as necessary for concurrent excision of bowel (eg G69.3 H11.1)
         *   Use supplementary code as necessary for relief of strangulation of bowel (eg G76.2 H17.5)*

T27.1   Repair of ventral hernia using insert of natural material
T27.2   Repair of ventral hernia using insert of prosthetic material
         Includes: Repair of ventral hernia using insert nec
T27.3   Repair of ventral hernia using sutures
T27.4   Removal of prosthetic material from previous repair of ventral hernia
T27.8   Other specified
T27.9   Unspecified

T28   **Other repair of anterior abdominal wall**
         Includes: Abdominal wall nec

T28.1   Closure of gastroschisis
         Includes: Closure of exomphalos
T28.2   Suture of anterior abdominal wall
         Includes: Suture of abdomen
         *   Closure of anterior abdominal wall*
         *   Closure of abdomen*
T28.3   Resuture of previous incision of anterior abdominal wall
         Includes: Resuture of rupture of incision of anterior abdominal wall
         *   Suture of dehiscence of wound of anterior abdominal wall*
T28.8   Other specified
T28.9   Unspecified

T29   **Operations on umbilicus**
Includes: Skin of umbilicus
Excludes: Repair of umbilical hernia (T24)
Note: Codes from Chapter S may be used to enhance these codes

T29.1   Excision of umbilicus
T29.2   Excision of urachus
Includes: Excision of lesion of urachus
T29.3   Extirpation of lesion of umbilicus
T29.4   Biopsy of lesion of umbilicus
Includes: Biopsy of umbilicus
T29.5   Excision of fistula of umbilicus
Includes: Excision of sinus of umbilicus
T29.6   Plastic operations on umbilicus
T29.8   Other specified
T29.9   Unspecified

T30   **Opening of abdomen**
Includes: Abdominal wall
*   Peritoneum*
*   Peritoneal cavity*
Note: Do not use as approach code (Y50)

T30.1   Reopening of abdomen and reexploration of intraabdominal operation site and surgical arrest of
postoperative bleeding
Includes: Reopening of incision of abdomen and reexploration of intraabdominal operation site and
*   surgical arrest of bleeding*
*   Reopening of wound of abdomen and reexploration of intraabdominal operation site and*
*   surgical arrest of bleeding*
T30.2   Reopening of abdomen and reexploration of intraabdominal operation site nec
Includes: Reopening of incision of abdomen and reexploration of intraabdominal operation site nec
*   Reopening of wound of abdomen and reexploration of intraabdominal operation site nec*
T30.3   Reopening of abdomen nec
Includes: Reopening of incision of abdomen nec
*   Reopening of wound of abdomen nec*
T30.8   Other specified
T30.9   Unspecified
Includes: Exploratory laparotomy nec

T31   **Other operations on anterior abdominal wall**
Includes: Abdominal wall nec

T31.1   Biopsy of lesion of anterior abdominal wall
Includes: Biopsy of anterior abdominal wall
T31.2   Excision of lesion of anterior abdominal wall and insert of prosthetic material into anterior abdominal
wall
T31.3   Excision of lesion of anterior abdominal wall nec
T31.4   Destruction of lesion of anterior abdominal wall
T31.5   Drainage of anterior abdominal wall
T31.6   Removal of foreign body from anterior abdominal wall
T31.8   Other specified
T31.9   Unspecified

T33   **Open extirpation of lesion of peritoneum**

T33.1   Open excision of lesion of peritoneum
T33.2   Open destruction of lesion of peritoneum
T33.8   Other specified
T33.9   Unspecified

T34   **Open drainage of peritoneum**
Excludes: Operations to create drainage into peritoneum (A12.4 A53)
           Creation of peritoneovenous shunt (L81.1)
           Peritoneal dialysis (X40.2)

T34.1   Open drainage of subphrenic abscess
T34.2   Open drainage of pelvic abscess
T34.3   Open drainage of abdominal abscess nec
T34.8   Other specified
T34.9   Unspecified

T36   **Operations on omentum**

T36.1   Omentectomy
T36.2   Excision of lesion of omentum
T36.3   Destruction of lesion of omentum
T36.4   Biopsy of lesion of omentum
         Includes: Biopsy of omentum
T36.5   Creation of omental flap
T36.8   Other specified
T36.9   Unspecified

T37   **Operations on mesentery of small intestine**

T37.1   Excision of lesion of mesentery of small intestine
T37.2   Destruction of lesion of mesentery of small intestine
T37.3   Biopsy of lesion of mesentery of small intestine
         Includes: Biopsy of mesentery of small intestine
                   Biopsy of lesion of mesentery nec
                   Biopsy of mesentery nec
T37.4   Repair of mesentery of small intestine
T37.8   Other specified
T37.9   Unspecified

T38   **Operations on mesentery of colon**

T38.1   Excision of lesion of mesentery of colon
T38.2   Destruction of lesion of mesentery of colon
T38.3   Biopsy of lesion of mesentery of colon
         Includes: Biopsy of mesentery of colon
T38.4   Repair of mesentery of colon
T38.8   Other specified
T38.9   Unspecified

T39   **Operations on posterior peritoneum**
           Includes: Posterior abdominal wall

T39.1   Excision of lesion of posterior peritoneum
T39.2   Destruction of lesion of posterior peritoneum
T39.3   Biopsy of lesion of posterior peritoneum
         Includes: Biopsy of posterior peritoneum
T39.8   Other specified
T39.9   Unspecified

T41   **Other open perations on peritoneum**
Includes: Peritoneal cavity

T41.1   Open biopsy of lesion of peritoneum nec
Includes: Open biopsy of peritoneum nec
        Biopsy of lesion of peritoneum nec
        Biopsy of peritoneum nec
T41.2   Division of band of peritoneum
T41.3   Freeing of adhesions of peritoneum
Includes: Freeing of adhesions of mesentery
        Freeing of adhesions of bowel
        Division of adhesions of peritoneum nec
        Division of adhesions of mesentery nec
        Division of adhesions of bowel nec
T41.4   Open removal of foreign body from peritoneum
Includes: Removal of foreign body from peritoneum nec
T41.8   Other specified
T41.9   Unspecified

T42   **Therapeutic endoscopic operations on peritoneum**
Includes: Peritoneal cavity
Note: *It is not necessary to code additionally any mention of diagnostic endoscopic examination of peritoneum (T43.9)*
        Therapeutic endoscopic operations specifically directed at individual intraabdominal organs are usually classified elsewhere

T42.1   Endoscopic resection of lesion of peritoneum
T42.2   Endoscopic destruction of lesion of peritoneum
T42.3   Endoscopic division of adhesions of peritoneum
Includes: Endoscopic division of adhesions of mesentery
        Endoscopic division of adhesions of bowel
T42.4   Endoscopic removal of foreign body from peritoneum
T42.8   Other specified
T42.9   Unspecified

T43   **Diagnostic endoscopic examination of peritoneum**
Includes: Peritoneal cavity
Note: *Diagnostic endoscopic examinations specifically directed at individual intraabdominal organs are usually classified elsewhere*

T43.1   Diagnostic endoscopic examination of peritoneum and biopsy of lesion of peritoneum
Includes: Diagnostic endoscopic examination of peritoneum and biopsy of peritoneum
        Endoscopic biopsy of lesion of peritoneum
        Endoscopic biopsy of peritoneum
T43.2   Diagnostic endoscopic examination of peritoneum and biopsy of lesion of intraabdominal organ nec
Includes: Diagnostic endoscopic examination of peritoneum and biopsy of intraabdominal organ nec
        Laparoscopic biopsy of lesion of intraabdominal organ nec
        Laparoscopic biopsy of intraabdominal organ nec
Note: *Use subsidiary site code as necessary*
T43.8   Other specified
T43.9   Unspecified
Includes: Gynaecological laparoscopy nec
        Laparoscopy nec
        Peritoneoscopy nec

T45   **Image controlled operations on abdominal cavity**

T45.1   Image controlled percutaneous drainage of subphrenic abscess
T45.2   Image controlled percutaneous drainage of pelvic abscess
T45.3   Image controlled percutaneous drainage of abdominal abscess nec
T45.8   Other specified
T45.9   Unspecified

T46 **Other drainage of peritoneal cavity**
Excludes: Operations to create drainage into peritoneum (A12.4 A53)
Creation of peritoneovenous shunt (L81.1)
Peritoneal dialysis (X40.2)

T46.1 Paracentesis abdominis for ascites
T46.2 Drainage of ascites nec
T46.3 Irrigation of peritoneal cavity
Includes: Lavage of peritoneal cavity
Washout of peritoneal cavity
T46.8 Other specified
T46.9 Unspecified

T48 **Other operations on peritoneum**
Includes: Peritoneal cavity

T48.1 Introduction of radioactive substance into peritoneal cavity
T48.2 Introduction of cytotoxic substance into peritoneal cavity
T48.3 Introduction of therapeutic substance into peritoneal cavity
T48.4 Introduction of substance into peritoneal cavity nec
T48.8 Other specified
T48.9 Unspecified

T50 **Transplantation of fascia**
Excludes: With skin (S18 S25)

T50.1 Transfer of fascial tissue
T50.8 Other specified
T50.9 Unspecified

T51 **Excision of fascia of abdomen**
Includes: Release of fascia of abdomen

T51.1 Excision of fascia of posterior abdominal wall
T51.2 Excision of fascia of pelvis
T51.8 Other specified
T51.9 Unspecified

T52 **Excision of other fascia**

T52.1 Palmar fasciectomy
T52.2 Revision of palmar fasciectomy
T52.3 Plantar fasciectomy
T52.4 Revision of plantar fasciectomy
T52.8 Other specified
T52.9 Unspecified
Includes: Fasciectomy nec

T53 **Extirpation of lesion of fascia**

T53.1 Excision of lesion of fascia
T53.2 Destruction of lesion of fascia
T53.8 Other specified
T53.9 Unspecified

T54 **Division of fascia**

T54.1 Division of palmar fascia
T54.2 Division of plantar fascia
T54.8 Other specified
T54.9 Unspecified
Includes: Fasciotomy nec

184

T55   Release of fascia
Excludes: Release of fascia of abdomen (T51)

T55.1   Release fasciotomy of upper arm
T55.2   Release fasciotomy of forearm
T55.3   Release fasciotomy of thigh
T55.4   Release fasciotomy of anterior compartment of lower leg
T55.5   Release fasciotomy of posterior compartment of lower leg
T55.6   Release fasciotomy of leg nec
T55.8   Other specified
T55.9   Unspecified

T57   Other operations on fascia

T57.1   Freeing of adhesions of fascia
T57.2   Biopsy of lesion of fascia
     Includes: Biopsy of fascia
T57.3   Repair of fascia
T57.4   Stripping of fascia
T57.8   Other specified
T57.9   Unspecified

T59   Excision of ganglion

T59.1   Excision of ganglion of wrist
T59.2   Excision of ganglion of hand nec
T59.3   Excision of ganglion of knee
T59.4   Excision of ganglion of foot
     Includes: Excision of ganglion of ankle
T59.8   Other specified
T59.9   Unspecified

T60   Reexcision of ganglion

T60.1   Reexcision of ganglion of wrist
T60.2   Reexcision of ganglion of hand nec
T60.3   Reexcision of ganglion of knee
T60.4   Reexcision of ganglion of foot
     Includes: Reexcision of ganglion of ankle
T60.8   Other specified
T60.9   Unspecified

T62   Operations on bursa

T62.1   Total excision of bursa
T62.2   Excision of bursa nec
T62.3   Biopsy of lesion of bursa
     Includes: Biopsy of bursa
T62.4   Aspiration of bursa
T62.5   Injection into bursa
T62.6   Exploration of bursa
T62.8   Other specified
T62.9   Unspecified

T64   Transposition of tendon

T64.1   Multiple transfer of tendon to tendon
T64.2   Transfer of tendon to tendon nec
T64.3   Multiple insertion of tendons into bone
T64.4   Insertion of tendon into bone nec
     Excludes: For stabilisation of joint (W77)
T64.5   Tenodesis
T64.8   Other specified
T64.9   Unspecified

T65   **Excision of tendon**

T65.1   Sacrifice of tendon
T65.2   Excision of lesion of tendon
T65.8   Other specified
T65.9   Unspecified

T67   **Primary repair of tendon**
        Includes: Repair of tendon nec

T67.1   Primary repair of tendon using tendon transfer procedure
T67.2   Primary repair of tendon using lengthening procedure
T67.3   Primary repair of tendon using permanent prosthesis
T67.4   Primary repair of tendon using temporary prosthesis
T67.5   Primary repair of tendon using graft
T67.6   Primary simple repair of tendon
        Includes: Primary end to end repair of tendon
T67.8   Other specified
T67.9   Unspecified

T68   **Secondary repair of tendon**

T68.1   Secondary repair of tendon using tendon transfer procedure
T68.2   Secondary repair of tendon using lengthening procedure
T68.3   Secondary repair of tendon using permanent prosthesis
T68.4   Secondary repair of tendon using temporary prosthesis
T68.5   Secondary repair of tendon using graft
T68.6   Secondary simple repair of tendon
        Includes: Secondary end to end repair of tendon
T68.8   Other specified
T68.9   Unspecified

T69   **Freeing of tendon**
        Excludes: For stabilisation of joint (W77)

T69.1   Primary tenolysis
T69.2   Revision of tenolysis
T69.8   Other specified
T69.9   Unspecified

T70   **Adjustment to length of tendon**

T70.1   Subcutaneous tenotomy
T70.2   Tenotomy nec
T70.3   Adjustment to muscle origin of tendon
T70.4   Shortening of tendon nec
T70.5   Lengthening of tendon
        Includes: Lengthening of muscle
T70.8   Other specified
T70.9   Unspecified

T71   **Excision of sheath of tendon**

T71.1   Tenosynovectomy
T71.8   Other specified
T71.9   Unspecified

T72   **Other operations on sheath of tendon**

T72.1   Reconstruction of sheath of tendon
T72.2   Biopsy of lesion of sheath of tendon
        Includes: Biopsy of sheath of tendon
T72.3   Release of constriction of sheath of tendon
T72.4   Exploration of sheath of tendon
T72.8   Other specified
T72.9   Unspecified

T74   **Other operations on tendon**

T74.1   Biopsy of lesion of tendon nec
        Includes: Biopsy of tendon nec
T74.2   Removal of prosthesis from tendon
T74.3   Exploration of tendon nec
T74.8   Other specified
T74.9   Unspecified

T76   **Transplantation of muscle**
        Excludes: With skin (S17 S24)

T76.1   Microvascular free tissue transfer of flap of muscle
T76.8   Other specified
T76.9   Unspecified

T77   **Excision of muscle**

T77.1   Excision of whole muscle group
T77.2   Wide excision of muscle
        Includes: Wide excision of lesion of muscle
T77.3   Partial excision of muscle nec
        Includes: Excision of lesion of muscle nec
                 Excision of Volkmann contracture of forearm
T77.4   Debridement of muscle nec
T77.8   Other specified
T77.9   Unspecified

T79   **Repair of muscle**

T79.1   Plastic repair of rotator cuff of shoulder
T79.2   Quadricepsplasty
T79.8   Other specified
T79.9   Unspecified

T80   **Release of contracture of muscle**

T80.1   Release of paralytic tether
T80.2   Release of cicatricial tether
T80.3   Release of webbing of neck
T80.4   Release of sternomastoid muscle
        Includes: Release of torticollis
T80.8   Other specified
T80.9   Unspecified

T81   **Biopsy of muscle**

T81.1   Percutaneous biopsy of muscle
        Includes: Percutaneous biopsy of lesion of muscle
        Note: *Use subsidiary code to identify method of image control as necessary (Y53)*
T81.2   Biopsy of neuromuscular junction
        Includes: Biopsy of muscle for biochemical study
                 Biopsy of muscle for physiological study
T81.3   Biopsy of lesion of muscle nec
T81.8   Other specified
T81.9   Unspecified

T83   **Other operations on muscle**

T83.1   Destruction of lesion of muscle
T83.2   Division of muscle nec
T83.3   Stretching of muscle
T83.4   Exploration of muscle
T83.8   Other specified
T83.9   Unspecified

T85   **Block dissection of lymph nodes**

T85.1   Block dissection of cervical lymph nodes
T85.2   Block dissection of axillary lymph nodes
T85.3   Block dissection of mediastinal lymph nodes
T85.4   Block dissection of paraaortic lymph nodes
T85.5   Block dissection of inguinal lymph nodes
T85.8   Other specified
T85.9   Unspecified

T86   **Sampling of lymph nodes**

T86.1   Sampling of cervical lymph nodes
T86.2   Sampling of axillary lymph nodes
T86.3   Sampling of supraclavicular lymph nodes
T86.4   Sampling of internal mammary lymph nodes
T86.5   Sampling of mediastinal lymph nodes
T86.6   Sampling of paraaortic lymph nodes
T86.7   Sampling of inguinal lymph nodes
T86.8   Other specified
T86.9   Unspecified

T87   **Excision or biopsy of lymph node**

T87.1   Excision or biopsy of scalene lymph node
T87.2   Excision or biopsy of cervical lymph node nec
T87.3   Excision or biopsy of axillary lymph node
        Includes: Excision or biopsy of supraclavicular lymph node
T87.4   Excision or biopsy of mediastinal lymph node
T87.5   Excision or biopsy of paraaortic lymph node
T87.6   Excision or biopsy of porta hepatis lymph node
T87.7   Excision or biopsy of inguinal lymph node
T87.8   Other specified
T87.9   Unspecified

T88   **Drainage of lesion of lymph node**

T88.1   Drainage of lesion of cervical lymph node
T88.2   Drainage of lesion of axillary lymph node
T88.3   Drainage of lesion of inguinal lymph node
T88.8   Other specified
T88.9   Unspecified

T89   **Operations on lymphatic duct**

T89.1   Reconstruction of lymphatic duct
T89.2   Bypass of obstruction of lymphatic duct
T89.3   Ligation of lymphatic duct
T89.4   Cannulation of lymphatic duct
T89.8   Other specified
T89.9   Unspecified

T90   **Contrast radiology of lymphatic tissue**

T90.1   Lymphangiography of arm
T90.2   Lymphangiography of mediastinal lymph nodes
T90.3   Lymphangiography of paraaortic lymph nodes
T90.4   Lymphangiography of leg
T90.8   Other specified
T90.9   Unspecified
        Includes: Lymphangiography nec

T92   **Other operations on lymphatic tissue**

T92.1   Excision of lymphocele
T92.2   Excision of lymphoedematous tissue of arm
T92.3   Excision of lymphoedematous tissue of leg and buried flaps hfq
T92.4   Excision of lymphoedematous tissue of leg nec
T92.5   Excision of lymphoedematous tissue of scrotum
T92.6   Excision of lymphoedematous tissue nec
T92.8   Other specified
T92.9   Unspecified

T94   **Operations on branchial cleft**

T94.1   Excision of branchial cyst
T94.2   Closure of branchial fistula
T94.8   Other specified
T94.9   Unspecified

T96   **Other operations on soft tissue**
         Includes: Connective tissue

T96.1   Excision of cystic hygroma
T96.2   Excision of lesion of soft tissue nec
T96.8   Other specified
T96.9   Unspecified

CHAPTER V

BONES AND JOINTS OF
SKULL AND SPINE

(CODES V01-V54)

Excludes: BONES AND JOINTS OF SACRUM AND COCCYX   (Chapter W)

V01   **Plastic repair of cranium**

V01.1   Cranioplasty using prosthesis
V01.2   Cranioplasty using bone graft
V01.3   Opening of suture of cranium
V01.4   Removal of prosthesis from cranium
V01.5   Revision of cranioplasty nec
V01.8   Other specified
V01.9   Unspecified

V03   **Opening of cranium**
        Note: *Do not use as approach code (Y46 Y47)*

V03.1   Exploratory open craniotomy
        Includes: Open craniotomy
V03.2   Reopening of cranium and reexploration of intracranial operation site and surgical arrest of postoperative bleeding
V03.3   Reopening of cranium and reexploration of intracranial operation site nec
V03.4   Reopening of cranium nec
V03.5   Trephine of cranium
V03.6   Exploratory burrhole of cranium
V03.8   Other specified
V03.9   Unspecified
        Includes: Exploratory craniotomy nec
                   Craniotomy nec

V05   **Other operations on cranium**

V05.1   Extirpation of lesion of cranium
V05.2   Biopsy of lesion of cranium
        Includes: Biopsy of cranium
V05.3   Elevation of depressed fracture of cranium
V05.4   Repair of fracture of cranium nec
V05.5   Graft of bone to cranium
V05.8   Other specified
V05.9   Unspecified

V07   **Excision of bone of face**

V07.1   Extensive excision of bone of face
V07.2   Partial excision of bone of face nec
V07.3   Excision of lesion of bone of face
        Excludes: Excision of dental lesion of maxilla (F18)
V07.8   Other specified
V07.9   Unspecified

V08   **Reduction of fracture of maxilla**

V08.1   Reduction of fracture of alveolus of maxilla
V08.2   Open reduction of fracture of maxilla nec
V08.3   Closed reduction of fracture of maxilla nec
V08.8   Other specified
V08.9   Unspecified

V09   Reduction of fracture of other bone of face

V09.1   Reduction of fracture of nasoethmoid complex of bones
V09.2   Reduction of fracture of nasal bone nec
         Includes: Reduction of fracture of nose
V09.3   Reduction of fracture of zygomatic complex of bones
V09.8   Other specified
V09.9   Unspecified

V10   Division of bone of face

V10.1   Intracranial osteotomy of bone of face
V10.2   Transorbital subcranial osteotomy of bone of face
V10.3   Osteotomy of maxilla involving nasal complex
V10.4   Low level osteotomy of maxilla
         Includes: Osteotomy of maxilla nec
V10.5   Osteotomy of alveolar segment of maxilla
         Includes: Dentoalveolar level osteotomy of maxilla
V10.8   Other specified
V10.9   Unspecified

V11   Fixation of bone of face
         Includes: Fixator of bone of face

V11.1   Intermaxillary fixation of maxilla
V11.2   Internal fixation of maxilla nec
V11.3   Extraoral fixation of maxilla
V11.4   Fixation of maxilla nec
V11.5   Removal of fixation from bone of face
V11.8   Other specified
V11.9   Unspecified

V13   Other operations on bone of face

V13.1   Reconstruction of bone of face
V13.2   Alveolar bone graft to maxilla
V13.3   Biopsy of lesion of bone of face
         Includes: Biopsy of bone of face
V13.8   Other specified
V13.9   Unspecified

V14   Excision of mandible
         Includes: Jaw nec

V14.1   Hemimandibulectomy
V14.2   Extensive excision of mandible nec
V14.3   Partial excision of mandible nec
         Includes: Limited excision of mandible nec
V14.4   Excision of lesion of mandible
         Excludes: Excision of dental lesion of mandible (F18)
V14.8   Other specified
V14.9   Unspecified
         Includes: Mandibulectomy nec

V15   Reduction of fracture of mandible
         Includes: Jaw nec

V15.1   Reduction of fracture of alveolus of mandible
V15.2   Open reduction of fracture of mandible nec
V15.3   Closed reduction of fracture of mandible nec
V15.8   Other specified
V15.9   Unspecified

V16   **Division of mandible**
Includes: Jaw nec

V16.1   Osteotomy of mandible and advancement of mandible
V16.2   Osteotomy of mandible and retrusion of mandible
V16.3   Osteotomy of alveolar segment of mandible
         Includes: Dentoalveolar level osteotomy of mandible
V16.8   Other specified
V16.9   Unspecified

V17   **Fixation of mandible**
Includes: Fixator of mandible
         Jaw nec

V17.1   Intermaxillary fixation of mandible
V17.2   Internal fixation of mandible nec
V17.3   Extraoral fixation of mandible
V17.4   Removal of fixation from mandible
V17.8   Other specified
V17.9   Unspecified

V19   **Other operations on mandible**
Includes: Jaw nec

V19.1   Reconstruction of mandible
V19.2   Genioplasty of mandible
V19.3   Alveolar bone graft to mandible
V19.4   Biopsy of lesion of mandible
         Includes: Biopsy of mandible
V19.5   Manipulation of mandible nec
V19.8   Other specified
V19.9   Unspecified

V20   **Reconstruction of temporomandibular joint**

V20.1   Total prosthetic replacement of temporomandibular joint
V20.2   Prosthetic replacement of temporomandibular joint nec
V20.3   Intraarticular arthroplasty of temporomandibular joint
V20.8   Other specified
V20.9   Unspecified
         Includes: Arthroplasty of temporomandibular joint nec

V21   **Other operations on temporomandibular joint**

V21.1   Meniscectomy of temporomandibular joint
V21.2   Reduction of dislocation of temporomandibular joint
V21.8   Other specified
V21.9   Unspecified

V22   **Primary decompression operations on cervical spine**
Includes: Decompression operations on cervical spine nec

V22.1   Primary anterior decompression of cervical spinal cord and fusion of joint of cervical spine
V22.2   Primary anterior decompression of cervical spinal cord nec
V22.3   Primary foraminotomy of cervical spine
V22.8   Other specified
V22.9   Unspecified

V23   **Revisional decompression operations on cervical spine**

V23.1   Revisional anterior decompression of cervical spinal cord and fusion of joint of cervical spine
V23.2   Revisional anterior decompression of cervical spinal cord nec
V23.3   Revisional foraminotomy of cervical spine
V23.8   Other specified
V23.9   Unspecified

V24   **Decompression operations on thoracic spine**

V24.1   Primary decompression of thoracic spinal cord and fusion of joint of thoracic spine
         Includes: Decompression of thoracic spinal cord and fusion of joint of thoracic spine
V24.2   Primary decompression of thoracic spinal cord nec
         Includes: Decompression of thoracic spinal cord nec
V24.3   Revisional decompression of thoracic spinal cord
V24.8   Other specified
V24.9   Unspecified

V25   **Primary decompression operations on lumbar spine**
         Includes: Decompression operations on lumbar spine nec

V25.1   Primary extended decompression of lumbar spinal cord and intertransverse fusion of joint of lumbar
         spine
V25.2   Primary extended decompression of lumbar spinal cord nec
V25.3   Primary posterior decompression of lumbar spinal cord and intertransverse fusion of joint of lumbar
         spine
V25.4   Primary posterior laminectomy decompression of lumbar spinal cord
V25.5   Primary posterior decompression of lumbar spinal cord nec
V25.6   Primary lateral foraminotomy of lumbar spine
V25.8   Other specified
V25.9   Unspecified

V26   **Revisional decompression operations on lumbar spine**

V26.1   Revisional extended decompression of lumbar spinal cord and intertransverse fusion of joint of lumbar
         spine
V26.2   Revisional extended decompression of lumbar spinal cord nec
V26.3   Revisional posterior decompression of lumbar spinal cord and intertransverse fusion of joint of lumbar
         spine
V26.4   Revisional posterior laminectomy decompression of lumbar spinal cord
V26.5   Revisional posterior decompression of lumbar spinal cord nec
V26.6   Revisional lateral foraminotomy of lumbar spine
V26.8   Other specified
V26.9   Unspecified

V27   **Decompression operations on unspecified spine**

V27.1   Primary decompression of spinal cord and fusion of joint of spine nec
         Includes: Decompression of spinal cord and fusion of joint of spine nec
V27.2   Primary decompression of spinal cord nec
         Includes: Decompression of spinal cord nec
V27.3   Revisional decompression of spinal cord nec
V27.8   Other specified
V27.9   Unspecified

V29   **Primary excision of cervical intervertebral disc**
         Includes: Excision of cervical intervertebral disc nec

V29.1   Primary laminectomy excision of cervical intervertebral disc
V29.2   Primary hemilaminectomy excision of cervical intervertebral disc
V29.3   Primary fenestration excision of cervical intervertebral disc
V29.4   Primary anterior excision of cervical intervertebral disc and interbody fusion of joint of cervical spine
V29.5   Primary anterior excision of cervical intervertebral disc nec
V29.6   Primary microdiscectomy of cervical intervertebral disc
V29.8   Other specified
V29.9   Unspecified

V30   **Revisional excision of cervical intervertebral disc**

V30.1   Revisional laminectomy excision of cervical intervertebral disc
V30.2   Revisional hemilaminectomy excision of cervical intervertebral disc
V30.3   Revisional fenestration excision of cervical intervertebral disc
V30.4   Revisional anterior excision of cervical intervertebral disc and interbody fusion of joint of cervical spine
V30.5   Revisional anterior excision of cervical intervertebral disc nec
V30.6   Revisional microdiscectomy of cervical intervertebral disc
V30.8   Other specified
V30.9   Unspecified

V31   **Primary excision of thoracic intervertebral disc**
       Includes: Excision of thoracic intervertebral disc nec

V31.1   Primary anterolateral excision of thoracic intervertebral disc and graft hfq
V31.2   Primary anterolateral excision of thoracic intervertebral disc nec
V31.3   Primary costotransversectomy of thoracic intervertebral disc
V31.8   Other specified
V31.9   Unspecified

V32   **Revisional excision of thoracic intervertebral disc**

V32.1   Revisional anterolateral excision of thoracic intervertebral disc and graft hfq
V32.2   Revisional anterolateral excision of thoracic intervertebral disc nec
V32.3   Revisional costotransversectomy of thoracic intervertebral disc
V32.8   Other specified
V32.9   Unspecified

V33   **Primary excision of lumbar intervertebral disc**
       Includes: Excision of lumbar intervertebral disc nec

V33.1   Primary laminectomy excision of lumbar intervertebral disc
V33.2   Primary fenestration excision of lumbar intervertebral disc
V33.3   Primary anterior excision of lumbar intervertebral disc and interbody fusion of joint of lumbar spine
V33.4   Primary anterior excision of lumbar intervertebral disc nec
V33.5   Primary anterior excision of lumbar intervertebral disc and posterior graft fusion of joint of lumbar spine
V33.6   Primary anterior excision of lumbar intervertebral disc and posterior instrumentation of lumbar spine
V33.7   Primary microdiscectomy of lumbar intervertebral disc
V33.8   Other specified
       Includes: Primary posterior excision of lumbar intervertebral disc
V33.9   Unspecified

V34   **Revisional excision of lumbar intervertebral disc**

V34.1   Revisional laminectomy excision of lumbar intervertebral disc
V34.2   Revisional fenestration excision of lumbar intervertebral disc
V34.3   Revisional anterior excision of lumbar intervertebral disc and interbody fusion of joint of lumbar spine
V34.4   Revisional anterior excision of lumbar intervertebral disc nec
V34.5   Revisional anterior excision of lumbar intervertebral disc and posterior graft fusion of joint of lumbar spine
V34.6   Revisional anterior excision of lumbar intervertebral disc and posterior instrumentation of lumbar spine
V34.7   Revisional microdiscectomy of lumbar intervertebral disc
V34.8   Other specified
       Includes: Revisional posterior excision of lumbar intervertebral disc
V34.9   Unspecified

V35   **Excision of unspecified intervertebral disc**

V35.1   Primary excision of intervertebral disc nec
       Includes: Excision of intervertebral disc nec
V35.2   Revisional excision of intervertebral disc nec
V35.8   Other specified
V35.9   Unspecified

V37   **Primary fusion of joint of cervical spine**
Includes: Fusion of joint of cervical spine nec

V37.1   Posterior fusion of atlantoaxial joint
V37.2   Posterior fusion of joint of cervical spine nec
V37.3   Transoral fusion of atlantoaxial joint
V37.4   Fusion of atlantooccipital joint
V37.8   Other specified
V37.9   Unspecified

V38   **Primary fusion of other joint of spine**
Includes: Fusion of joint of spine nec
Unspecified spine

V38.1   Primary fusion of joint of thoracic spine
V38.2   Primary posterior interlaminar fusion of joint of lumbar spine
V38.3   Primary posterior fusion of joint of lumbar spine nec
       Includes: Primary posterior interspinous fusion of lumbar spine
V38.4   Primary intertransverse fusion of joint of lumbar spine nec
V38.8   Other specified
V38.9   Unspecified

V39   **Revisional fusion of joint of spine**

V39.1   Revisional fusion of joint of cervical spine
V39.2   Revisional fusion of joint of thoracic spine
V39.3   Revisional posterior interlaminar fusion of joint of lumbar spine
V39.4   Revisional posterior fusion of joint of lumbar spine nec
       Includes: Revisional posterior interspinous fusion of lumbar spine
V39.5   Revisional intertransverse fusion of joint of lumbar spine nec
V39.8   Other specified
V39.9   Unspecified

V41   **Instrumental correction of deformity of spine**

V41.1   Posterior attachment of correctional instrument to spine
V41.2   Anterior attachment of correctional instrument to spine
V41.3   Removal of correctional instrument from spine
V41.8   Other specified
V41.9   Unspecified

V42   **Other correction of deformity of spine**

V42.1   Excision of rib hump
V42.2   Epiphysiodesis of spinal apophyseal joint for correction of deformity
V42.3   Anterolateral release of spine for correction of deformity and graft hfq
V42.8   Other specified
V42.9   Unspecified

V43   **Extirpation of lesion of spine**

V43.1   Excision of lesion of cervical vertebra
V43.2   Excision of lesion of thoracic vertebra
V43.3   Excision of lesion of lumbar vertebra
V43.8   Other specified
V43.9   Unspecified

V44   **Decompression of fracture of spine**

V44.1   Complex decompression of fracture of spine
V44.2   Anterior decompression of fracture of spine
V44.3   Posterior decompression of fracture of spine
V44.8   Other specified
V44.9   Unspecified

V45   Other reduction of fracture of spine

V45.1   Open reduction of fracture of spine and excision of facet of spine
V45.2   Open reduction of fracture of spine nec
V45.3   Manipulative reduction of fracture of spine
V45.8   Other specified
V45.9   Unspecified

V46   Fixation of fracture of spine

V46.1   Fixation of fracture of spine using plate
V46.2   Fixation of fracture of spine using Harrington rod
V46.3   Fixation of fracture of spine using wire
V46.4   Fixation of fracture of spine and skull traction hfq
V46.8   Other specified
V46.9   Unspecified

V47   Biopsy of spine
Includes: Biopsy of lesion of spine

V47.1   Biopsy of cervical vertebra
V47.2   Biopsy of thoracic vertebra
V47.3   Biopsy of lumbar vertebra
V47.8   Other specified
V47.9   Unspecified

V48   Denervation of spinal facet joint of vertebra

V48.1   Radiofrequency controlled thermal denervation of spinal facet joint of cervical vertebra
V48.2   Denervation of spinal facet joint of cervical vertebra nec
V48.3   Radiofrequency controlled thermal denervation of spinal facet joint of thoracic vertebra
V48.4   Denervation of spinal facet joint of thoracic vertebra nec
V48.5   Radiofrequency controlled thermal denervation of spinal facet joint of lumbar vertebra
V48.6   Denervation of spinal facet joint of lumbar vertebra nec
V48.7   Radiofrequency controlled thermal denervation of spinal facet joint of vertebra nec
V48.8   Other specified
V48.9   Unspecified

V49   Exploration of spine
Note: Do not use as approach code (Y48-Y50)

V49.1   Exploratory cervical laminectomy
V49.2   Exploratory thoracic laminectomy
V49.3   Exploratory lumbar laminectomy
V49.4   Exploratory laminectomy nec
V49.5   Transthoracic exploration of spine
V49.6   Transperitoneal exploration of spine
V49.8   Other specified
V49.9   Unspecified

V50   Manipulation of spine

V50.1   Manipulation of spine using traction
V50.8   Other specified
V50.9   Unspecified

V52   Other operations on intervertebral disc

V52.1   Enzyme destruction of intervertebral disc
V52.2   Destruction of intervertebral disc nec
V52.3   Discography of intervertebral disc
V52.4   Biopsy of lesion of intervertebral disc nec
        Includes: Biopsy of intervertebral disc nec
V52.8   Other specified
V52.9   Unspecified

V54   Other operations on spine

V54.1   Transoral excision of odontoid process of axis
V54.2   Graft of bone to spine nec
V54.3   Osteotomy of spine nec
V54.4   Injection around spinal facet of spine
V54.8   Other specified
V54.9   Unspecified

CHAPTER W

OTHER BONES AND JOINTS

(CODES W01-W92)

Excludes: SOME OPERATIONS ON BONES FOR CORRECTION OF
CONGENITAL DEFORMITY OF LIMB   (Chapter X)

W01   **Complex reconstruction of thumb**
       Excludes: Some similar operations for correction of congenital deformity (X19-X27)

W01.1   Microvascular transfer of toe to thumb
W01.2   Pollicisation of finger
W01.3   Reconstruction of thumb using bone graft and skin flap
W01.4   Reconstruction of thumb using bone lengthening procedure
W01.5   Opposition transfer to thumb
W01.8   Other specified
W01.9   Unspecified

W02   **Other complex reconstruction of hand**
       Excludes: Some similar operations for correction of congenital deformity (X19-X27)

W02.1   Proximal row carpectomy
W02.2   Metacarpal support operations on carpus
W02.3   Multiple joint reconstruction of hand nec
W02.4   Complex reconstruction of soft tissue of hand nec
W02.8   Other specified
W02.9   Unspecified

W03   **Complex reconstruction of forefoot**
       Excludes: Some similar operations for correction of congenital deformity (X19-X27)

W03.1   Excision of heads of multiple lesser metatarsals
W03.2   Osteotomy of multiple metatarsals
W03.3   Total correction of claw toe
W03.4   Transfer of extensor hallucis longus tendon to head of first metatarsal head and fusion of interphalangeal joints
W03.5   Localised fusion of joints of midfoot and forefoot
W03.8   Other specified
W03.9   Unspecified

W04   **Complex reconstruction of hindfoot**
       Excludes: Some similar operations for correction of congenital deformity (X19-X27)

W04.1   Localised fusion of joints of hindfoot
W04.2   Triple fusion of joints of hindfoot
W04.3   Subtalar fusion of joints of hindfoot
W04.4   Stripping of muscle from os calcis
W04.5   Release of medial soft tissue of hindfoot and excision of lateral wedge of os calcis and fusion of os calcis
W04.8   Other specified
W04.9   Unspecified

W05   **Prosthetic replacement of bone**
       Excludes: Prosthetic replacement of joint (W37-W55)

W05.1   Articulated prosthetic replacement of bone
W05.8   Other specified
W05.9   Unspecified

W06   **Total excision of bone**
Excludes: Excision of rib to gain access to chest cavity (T03.9)

W06.1   Total excision of cervical rib
W06.2   Total excision of rib nec
W06.3   Total excision of patella
W06.4   Total excision of sesamoid bone nec
W06.5   Total excision of bone of foot nec
W06.6   Total excision of coccyx
W06.8   Other specified
W06.9   Unspecified
Includes: Ostectomy nec

W07   **Excision of ectopic bone**

W07.1   Excision of cross union of bone
W07.2   Excision of periarticular ectopic bone
W07.3   Excision of intramuscular ectopic bone
W07.8   Other specified
W07.9   Unspecified

W08   **Other excision of bone**
Excludes: For complex reconstruction of foot (W03-W04)
Some similar operations for correction of congenital deformity (X19-X27)

W08.1   Excision of natural protuberance of bone
Includes: Excision of tuberosity of bone
Excision of tubercle of bone
W08.2   Excision of overgrowth of bone
W08.3   Excision of excrescence of bone
W08.4   Excision of fragment of bone
W08.5   Partial excision of bone nec
W08.8   Other specified
W08.9   Unspecified

W09   **Extirpation of lesion of bone**

W09.1   Excision of lesion of bone
W09.2   Curettage of lesion of bone and graft hfq
W09.3   Curettage of lesion of bone nec
W09.4   Destruction of lesion of bone nec
W09.8   Other specified
W09.9   Unspecified

W10   **Open surgical fracture of bone**

W10.1   Open osteoclasis and angular correction and internal fixation hfq
W10.2   Open osteoclasis and angular correction and external fixation hfq
W10.3   Open osteoclasis and angular correction nec
W10.4   Open osteoclasis and internal fixation nec
W10.5   Open osteoclasis and external fixation nec
W10.8   Other specified
W10.9   Unspecified
Includes: Open osteoclasis nec

W11   **Other surgical fracture of bone**

W11.1   Closed osteoclasis
W11.8   Other specified
W11.9   Unspecified

W12 **Angulation periarticular division of bone**
Excludes: For stabilisation of joint (W77.5)
Some similar operations for correction of congenital deformity (X19-X27)

W12.1 Biosseus angulation periarticular osteotomy and internal fixation hfq
W12.2 Angulation periarticular osteotomy and internal fixation nec
W12.3 Biosseus angulation periarticular osteotomy and external fixation hfq
W12.4 Angulation periarticular osteotomy and external fixation nec
W12.5 Biosseus angulation periarticular osteotomy nec
W12.8 Other specified
W12.9 Unspecified
Includes: Angulation periarticular osteotomy nec

W13 **Other periarticular division of bone**
Excludes: For stabilisation of joint (W77.5)
Some similar operations for correction of congenital deformity (X19-X27)

W13.1 Rotation periarticular osteotomy
W13.2 Displacement osteotomy
W13.3 Cuneiform osteotomy
W13.8 Other specified
W13.9 Unspecified

W14 **Diaphyseal division of bone**

W14.1 Angulation diaphyseal osteotomy and internal fixation hfq
W14.2 Angulation diaphyseal osteotomy and external fixation hfq
W14.3 Angulation diaphyseal osteotomy nec
W14.4 Rotation diaphyseal osteotomy and internal fixation hfq
W14.5 Rotation diaphyseal osteotomy and external fixation hfq
W14.6 Rotation diaphyseal osteotomy nec
W14.8 Other specified
W14.9 Unspecified

W15 **Division of bone of foot**
Excludes: For complex reconstruction of foot (W03-W04)
Some similar operations for correction of congenital deformity (X19-X27)
Note: **Use as secondary code when associated with soft tissue correction of hallux valgus (W79.1)**

W15.1 Osteotomy of neck of first metatarsal bone
W15.2 Osteotomy of base of first metatarsal bone
W15.3 Osteotomy of first metatarsal bone nec
W15.4 Osteotomy of head of metatarsal bone
W15.5 Osteotomy of midfoot tarsal bone
W15.8 Other specified
W15.9 Unspecified

W16 **Other division of bone**
Excludes: Some similar operations for correction of congenital deformity (X19-X27)

W16.1 Multiple osteotomy and internal fixation hfq
W16.2 Multiple osteotomy and external fixation hfq
W16.3 Multiple osteotomy nec
W16.4 Osteotomy and internal fixation nec
W16.5 Osteotomy and external fixation nec
W16.8 Other specified
W16.9 Unspecified
Includes: Osteotomy nec

W17   Other reconstruction of bone
Excludes: Some similar operations for correction of congenital deformity (X19-X27)

W17.1   Step cut lengthening of bone
W17.2   Traction lengthening of diaphysis of bone
W17.3   Traction lengthening of epiphyseal plate of bone
W17.4   Shortening of bone
W17.5   Revision of reconstruction of bone
W17.8   Other specified
W17.9   Unspecified

W18   Drainage of bone

W18.1   Fenestration of cortex of bone
W18.2   Saucerisation of bone
W18.3   Sequestrectomy of bone
W18.4   Decompression of fourage of bone
W18.5   Insertion of drainage system into bone
W18.6   Removal of drainage system from bone
W18.8   Other specified
W18.9   Unspecified

W19   Primary open reduction of fracture of bone and intramedullary fixation
Includes: Open reduction of fracture of bone and intramedullary fixation
Excludes: Fracture dislocation (W65)

W19.1   Primary open reduction of fracture of neck of femur and open fixation using pin and plate
        *Includes: Primary open reduction of fracture of neck of femur and open fixation using dynamic hip
                  screw*
W19.2   Primary open reduction of fracture of long bone and fixation using rigid nail nec
W19.3   Primary open reduction of fracture of long bone and fixation using flexible nail
W19.4   Primary open reduction of fracture of small bone and fixation using screw
W19.5   Primary open reduction of fragment of bone and fixation using screw
W19.6   Primary open reduction of fragment of bone and fixation using wire system
W19.8   Other specified
W19.9   Unspecified

W20   Primary open reduction of fracture of bone and extramedullary fixation
Includes: Primary open reduction of fracture of bone and fixation nec
*   Open reduction of fracture of bone and extramedullary fixation*
*   Open reduction of fracture of bone and fixation nec*
Excludes: Fracture dislocation (W65)

W20.1   Primary open reduction of fracture of long bone and extramedullary fixation using plate nec
W20.2   Primary open reduction of fracture of long bone and extramedullary fixation using circlage
W20.3   Primary open reduction of fracture of long bone and extramedullary fixation using suture
W20.4   Primary open reduction of fracture of long bone and complex extramedullary fixation nec
W20.5   Primary open reduction of fracture of ankle and extramedullary fixation nec
W20.6   Wiring of sternum
W20.8   Other specified
W20.9   Unspecified

W21   Primary open reduction of intraarticular fracture of bone
Includes: Open reduction of intraarticular fracture of bone
Excludes: Fracture dislocation (W65)

W21.1   Primary reduction of intraarticular fracture of bone using arthrotomy as approach
W21.2   Primary excision of intraarticular fragment of intraarticular fracture of bone
W21.3   Primary fixation of fragment of chondral cartilage of intraarticular fracture of bone
W21.4   Primary intraarticular fixation of intraarticular fracture of bone nec
W21.5   Primary extraarticular reduction of intraarticular fracture of bone
W21.8   Other specified
W21.9   Unspecified

W22 **Other primary open reduction of fracture of bone**
Includes: Open reduction of fracture of bone nec
Excludes   Fracture dislocation (W65)

W22.1 Primary open reduction of fracture of bone and skeletal traction hfq
W22.2 Primary open reduction of fracture of bone and external fixation hfq
W22.8 Other specified
W22.9 Unspecified

W23 **Secondary open reduction of fracture of bone**

W23.1 Secondary open reduction of fracture of bone and intramedullary fixation hfq
W23.2 Secondary open reduction of fracture of bone and extramedullary fixation hfq
W23.3 Secondary open reduction of intraarticular fracture of bone
W23.4 Secondary open reduction of fracture of bone and skeletal traction hfq
W23.5 Secondary open reduction of fracture of bone and external fixation hfq
W23.8 Other specified
W23.9 Unspecified

W24 **Closed reduction of fracture of bone and internal fixation**
Includes: Internal fixation of fracture of bone without mention of reduction
Excludes: Fracture dislocation (W66)

W24.1 Closed reduction of intracapsular fracture of neck of femur and fixation using nail or screw
W24.2 Closed reduction of fracture of long bone and rigid internal fixation nec
W24.3 Closed reduction of fracture of long bone and flexible internal fixation hfq
W24.4 Closed reduction of fracture of small bone and fixation using screw
W24.5 Closed reduction of fragment of bone and fixation using screw
W24.8 Other specified
W24.9 Unspecified

W25 **Closed reduction of fracture of bone and external fixation**
Includes: External fixation of fracture of bone without mention of reduction
Excludes: Fracture dislocation (W66)

W25.1 Closed reduction of fracture of bone and fixation to skeleton hfq
W25.2 Closed reduction of fracture of bone and fixation using functional bracing system
Includes: Closed reduction of fracture of bone and fixation using cast brace
W25.3 Remanipulation of fracture of bone and external fixation hfq
W25.8 Other specified
W25.9 Unspecified

W26 **Other closed reduction of fracture of bone**
Excludes: Fracture dislocation (W66)

W26.1 Manipulation of fracture of bone and skeletal traction nec
W26.2 Manipulation of fracture of bone nec
W26.3 Remanipulation of fracture of bone and skeletal traction nec
W26.4 Remanipulation of fracture of bone nec
W26.8 Other specified
W26.9 Unspecified

W27 **Fixation of epiphysis**

W27.1 Permanent cross union epiphysiodesis
W27.2 Epiphysioplasty
W27.3 Insertion of staple into epiphysis
W27.4 Removal of staple from epiphysis
W27.5 Temporary fixation of epiphysis
W27.8 Other specified
W27.9 Unspecified
Includes: Epiphysiodesis nec

W28   **Other internal fixation of bone**
Includes: Internal fixator of bone nec

W28.1   Application of internal fixation to bone nec
W28.2   Adjustment to internal fixation of bone nec
W28.3   Removal of internal fixation from bone nec
W28.8   Other specified
W28.9   Unspecified

W29   **Skeletal traction of bone**

W29.1   Application of skeletal traction to bone nec
W29.2   Adjustment to skeletal traction of bone
W29.3   Removal of skeletal traction from bone
W29.8   Other specified
W29.9   Unspecified

W30   **Other external fixation of bone**
Includes: External fixator of bone nec
         Fixation of bone nec
         Fixator of bone nec
Excludes: Immobilisation (X48-X49)

W30.1   Application of external fixation to bone nec
W30.2   Adjustment to external fixation of bone nec
W30.3   Removal of external fixation from bone nec
W30.8   Other specified
W30.9   Unspecified

W31   **Other autograft of bone**
Excludes: Autograft of bone marrow (W34.1)

W31.1   Inlay autograft to cortex of bone
W31.2   Onlay autograft to cortex of bone
W31.3   Cancellous strip autograft of bone
W31.4   Cancellous chip autograft of bone
W31.8   Other specified
W31.9   Unspecified

W32   **Other graft of bone**

W32.1   Prepared graft of bone
W32.2   Allograft of bone nec
         Excludes: Allograft of bone marrow nec (W34.2)
W32.3   Xenograft of bone
W32.8   Other specified
W32.9   Unspecified

W33   **Other open operations on bone**
Excludes: Some similar operations for correction of congenital deformity (X19-X27)

W33.1   Open biopsy of lesion of bone
         Includes: Open biopsy of bone
W33.2   Debridement of open fracture of bone
W33.3   Suture of periosteum
W33.4   Implantation of electromagnetic stimulator into bone
W33.5   Attention to electromagnetic stimulator in bone
W33.8   Other specified
W33.9   Unspecified

W34 Graft of bone marrow

W34.1 Autograft of bone marrow
W34.2 Allograft of bone marrow nec
W34.8 Other specified
W34.9 Unspecified

W35 Therapeutic puncture of bone
Note: Use subsidiary code to identify method of image control as necessary (Y53)

W35.1 Introduction of therapeutic substance into bone
W35.2 Introduction of destructive substance into bone
W35.3 Removal of implanted substance from bone
W35.4 Therapeutic drilling of bone nec
W35.5 Therapeutic percutaneous puncture of bone
W35.8 Other specified
W35.9 Unspecified

W36 Diagnostic puncture of bone
Note: Use subsidiary code to identify method of image control as necessary (Y53)

W36.1 Percutaneous needle biopsy of lesion of bone
    Includes: Percutaneous needle biopsy of bone
W36.2 Needle biopsy of lesion of bone nec
    Includes: Needle biopsy of bone nec
            Biopsy of lesion of bone nec
            Biopsy of bone nec
W36.3 Diagnostic drilling of bone
W36.4 Diagnostic puncture of sternum
    Includes: Aspiration of bone marrow of sternum
W36.5 Diagnostic extraction of bone marrow nec
    Includes: Aspiration of bone marrow nec
W36.8 Other specified
W36.9 Unspecified

W37 Total prosthetic replacement of hip joint using cement

W37.1 Primary total prosthetic replacement of hip joint using cement
W37.2 Conversion to total prosthetic replacement of hip joint using cement
    Note: Use subsidiary conversion from code as necessary
W37.3 Revision of total prosthetic replacement of hip joint using cement
W37.8 Other specified
W37.9 Unspecified
W37.0 Conversion from previous cemented total prosthetic replacement of hip joint

W38 Total prosthetic replacement of hip joint not using cement

W38.1 Primary total prosthetic replacement of hip joint not using cement
W38.2 Conversion to total prosthetic replacement of hip joint not using cement
    Note: Use subsidiary conversion from code as necessary
W38.3 Revision of total prosthetic replacement of hip joint not using cement
W38.8 Other specified
W38.9 Unspecified
W38.0 Conversion from previous uncemented total prosthetic replacement of hip joint

W39 Other total prosthetic replacement of hip joint

W39.1 Primary total prosthetic replacement of hip joint nec
W39.2 Conversion to total prosthetic replacement of hip joint nec
    Note: Use subsidiary conversion from code as necessary
W39.3 Revision of total prosthetic replacement of hip joint nec
W39.4 Attention to total prosthetic replacement of hip joint nec
W39.8 Other specified
W39.9 Unspecified
W39.0 Conversion from previous total prosthetic replacement of hip joint nec

W40   **Total prosthetic replacement of knee joint using cement**

W40.1   Primary total prosthetic replacement of knee joint using cement
W40.2   Conversion to total prosthetic replacement of knee joint using cement
        Note: *Use subsidiary conversion from code as necessary*
W40.3   Revision of total prosthetic replacement of knee joint using cement
W40.8   Other specified
W40.9   Unspecified
W40.0   Conversion from previous cemented total prosthetic replacement of knee joint

W41   **Total prosthetic replacement of knee joint not using cement**

W41.1   Primary total prosthetic replacement of knee joint not using cement
W41.2   Conversion to total prosthetic replacement of knee joint not using cement
        Note: *Use subsidiary conversion from code as necessary*
W41.3   Revision of total prosthetic replacement of knee joint not using cement
W41.8   Other specified
W41.9   Unspecified
W41.0   Conversion from previous uncemented total prosthetic replacement of knee joint

W42   **Other total prosthetic replacement of knee joint**

W42.1   Primary total prosthetic replacement of knee joint nec
W42.2   Conversion to total prosthetic replacement of knee joint nec
        Note: *Use subsidiary conversion from code as necessary*
W42.3   Revision of total prosthetic replacement of knee joint nec
W42.4   Attention to total prosthetic replacement of knee joint nec
W42.8   Other specified
W42.9   Unspecified
W42.0   Conversion from previous total prosthetic replacement of knee joint nec

W43   **Total prosthetic replacement of other joint using cement**

W43.1   Primary total prosthetic replacement of joint using cement nec
W43.2   Conversion to total prosthetic replacement of joint using cement nec
        Note: *Use subsidiary conversion from code as necessary*
W43.3   Revision of total prosthetic replacement of joint using cement nec
W43.8   Other specified
W43.9   Unspecified
W43.0   Conversion from previous cemented total prosthetic replacement of joint nec

W44   **Total prosthetic replacement of other joint not using cement**

W44.1   Primary total prosthetic replacement of joint not using cement nec
W44.2   Conversion to total prosthetic replacement of joint not using cement nec
        Note: *Use subsidiary conversion from code as necessary*
W44.3   Revision of total prosthetic replacement of joint not using cement nec
W44.8   Other specified
W44.9   Unspecified
W44.0   Conversion from previous uncemented total prosthetic replacement of joint nec

W45   **Other total prosthetic replacement of other joint**

W45.1   Primary total prosthetic replacement of joint nec
W45.2   Conversion to total prosthetic replacement of joint nec
        Note: *Use subsidiary conversion from code as necessary*
W45.3   Revision of total prosthetic replacement of joint nec
W45.4   Attention to total prosthetic replacement of joint nec
W45.8   Other specified
W45.9   Unspecified
W45.0   Conversion from previous total prosthetic replacement of joint nec

W46   Prosthetic replacement of head of femur using cement
Includes: Prosthetic hemiarthroplasty of head of femur using cement

W46.1   Primary prosthetic replacement of head of femur using cement
W46.2   Conversion to prosthetic replacement of head of femur using cement
         Note: Use subsidiary conversion from code as necessary
W46.3   Revision of prosthetic replacement of head of femur using cement
W46.8   Other specified
W46.9   Unspecified
W46.0   Conversion from previous cemented prosthetic replacement of head of femur

W47   Prosthetic replacement of head of femur not using cement
Includes: Prosthetic hemiarthroplasty of head of femur not using cement

W47.1   Primary prosthetic replacement of head of femur not using cement
W47.2   Conversion to prosthetic replacement of head of femur not using cement
         Note: Use subsidiary conversion from code as necessary
W47.3   Revision of prosthetic replacement of head of femur not using cement
W47.8   Other specified
W47.9   Unspecified
W47.0   Conversion from previous uncemented prosthetic replacement of head of femur

W48   Other prosthetic replacement of head of femur
Includes: Prosthetic hemiarthroplasty of head of femur nec

W48.1   Primary prosthetic replacement of head of femur nec
W48.2   Conversion to prosthetic replacement of head of femur nec
         Note: Use subsidiary conversion from code as necessary
W48.3   Revision of prosthetic replacement of head of femur nec
W48.4   Attention to prosthetic replacement of head of femur nec
W48.8   Other specified
W48.9   Unspecified
W48.0   Conversion from previous prosthetic replacement of head of femur nec

W49   Prosthetic replacement of head of humerus using cement
Includes: Prosthetic hemiarthroplasty of head of humerus using cement

W49.1   Primary prosthetic replacement of head of humerus using cement
W49.2   Conversion to prosthetic replacement of head of humerus using cement
         Note: Use subsidiary conversion from code as necessary
W49.3   Revision of prosthetic replacement of head of humerus using cement
W49.8   Other specified
W49.9   Unspecified
W49.0   Conversion from previous cemented prosthetic replacement of head of humerus

W50   Prosthetic replacement of head of humerus not using cement
Includes: Prosthetic hemiarthroplasty of head of humerus not using cement

W50.1   Primary prosthetic replacement of head of humerus not using cement
W50.2   Conversion to prosthetic replacement of head of humerus not using cement
         Note: Use subsidiary conversion from code as necessary
W50.3   Revision of prosthetic replacement of head of humerus not using cement
W50.8   Other specified
W50.9   Unspecified
W50.0   Conversion from previous uncemented prosthetic replacement of head of humerus

W51   Other prosthetic replacement of head of humerus
Includes: Prosthetic hemiarthroplasty of head of humerus nec

W51.1   Primary prosthetic replacement of head of humerus nec
W51.2   Conversion to prosthetic replacement of head of humerus nec
         Note: Use subsidiary conversion from code as necessary
W51.3   Revision of prosthetic replacement of head of humerus nec
W51.4   Attention to prosthetic replacement of head of humerus nec
W51.8   Other specified
W51.9   Unspecified
W51.0   Conversion from previous prosthetic replacement of head of humerus nec

W52   **Prosthetic replacement of articulation of other bone using cement**
Includes: Prosthetic hemiarthroplasty of articulation of bone using cement nec

W52.1   Primary prosthetic replacement of articulation of bone using cement nec
W52.2   Conversion to prosthetic replacement of articulation of bone using cement nec
         Note: Use subsidiary conversion from code as necessary
W52.3   Revision of prosthetic replacement of articulation of bone using cement nec
W52.8   Other specified
W52.9   Unspecified
W52.0   Conversion from previous cemented prosthetic replacement of articulation of bone nec

W53   **Prosthetic replacement of articulation of other bone not using cement**
Includes: Prosthetic hemiarthroplasty of articulation of bone not using cement nec

W53.1   Primary prosthetic replacement of articulation of bone not using cement nec
W53.2   Conversion to prosthetic replacement of articulation of bone not using cement nec
         Note: Use subsidiary conversion from code as necessary
W53.3   Revision of prosthetic replacement of articulation of bone not using cement nec
W53.8   Other specified
W53.9   Unspecified
W53.0   Conversion from previous uncemented prosthetic replacement of articulation of bone nec

W54   **Other prosthetic replacement of articulation of other bone**
Includes: Prosthetic hemiarthroplasty of articulation of bone nec

W54.1   Primary prosthetic replacement of articulation of bone nec
W54.2   Conversion to prosthetic replacement of articulation of bone nec
         Note: Use subsidiary conversion from code as necessary
W54.3   Revision of prosthetic replacement of articulation of bone nec
W54.4   Attention to prosthetic replacement of articulation of bone nec
W54.8   Other specified
W54.9   Unspecified
W54.0   Conversion from previous prosthetic replacement of articulation of bone nec

W55   **Prosthetic interposition reconstruction of joint**
Excludes: Some similar operations for correction of congenital deformity (X19-X27)

W55.1   Primary prosthetic interposition arthroplasty of joint
         Includes: Prosthetic interposition arthroplasty of joint
W55.2   Revision of prosthetic interposition arthroplasty of joint
W55.3   Conversion to prosthetic interposition arthroplasty of joint
         Note: Use subsidiary conversion from code as necessary
W55.4   Attention to prosthetic interposition arthroplasty of joint nec
W55.8   Other specified
W55.9   Unspecified
W55.0   Conversion from previous prosthetic interposition arthroplasty of joint

W56   **Other interposition reconstruction of joint**
Includes: Interposition reconstruction of joint using natural tissue
Excludes: Some similar operations for correction of congenital deformity (X19-X27)

W56.1   Primary interposition arthroplasty of metatarsophalangeal joint nec
         Includes: Interposition arthroplasty of metatarsophalangeal joint nec
W56.2   Primary interposition arthroplasty of joint nec
         Includes: Interposition arthroplasty of joint nec
W56.3   Revision of interposition arthroplasty of joint nec
W56.4   Conversion to interposition arthroplasty of joint nec
         Note: Use subsidiary conversion from code as necessary
W56.8   Other specified
W56.9   Unspecified
W56.0   Conversion from previous interposition arthroplasty of joint nec

W57 Excision reconstruction of joint
Excludes: *Some similar operations for correction of congenital deformity (X19-X27)*

W57.1 Primary excision arthroplasty of first metatarsophalangeal joint
Includes: *Excision arthroplasty of first metatarsophalangeal joint*
W57.2 Primary excision arthroplasty of joint nec
Includes: *Excision arthroplasty of joint nec*
W57.3 Revision of excision arthroplasty of joint
W57.4 Conversion to excision arthroplasty of joint
Note: *Use subsidiary conversion from code as necessary*
W57.8 Other specified
W57.9 Unspecified
W57.0 Conversion from previous excision arthroplasty of joint

W58 Other reconstruction of joint
Excludes: *Some similar operations for correction of congenital deformity (X19-X27)*

W58.1 Primary resurfacing arthroplasty of joint
W58.2 Revision of resurfacing arthroplasty of joint
W58.8 Other specified
W58.9 Unspecified
W58.0 Conversion from previous resurfacing arthroplasty of joint

W59 Fusion of joint of toe
Excludes: *For complex reconstruction of foot (W03-W04)*
Note: *Use as secondary code when associated with soft tissue correction of hallux valgus (W79.1)*

W59.1 Fusion of first metatarsophalangeal joint and replacement of lesser metatarsophalangeal joint
W59.2 Fusion of first metatarsophalangeal joint and excision of lesser metatarsophalangeal joint
W59.3 Fusion of first metatarsophalangeal joint nec
W59.4 Fusion of interphalangeal joint of great toe
W59.5 Fusion of interphalangeal joint of toe nec
W59.6 Revision of fusion of joint of toe
W59.8 Other specified
W59.9 Unspecified

W60 Fusion of other joint and extraarticular bone graft
Includes: *Fusion of joint and bone graft nec*

W60.1 Primary arthrodesis and extraarticular bone graft nec
Includes: *Arthrodesis and extraarticular bone graft nec*
W60.2 Revision of arthrodesis and extraarticular bone graft nec
W60.3 Conversion to arthrodesis and extraarticular bone graft nec
Note: *Use subsidiary conversion from code as necessary*
W60.8 Other specified
W60.9 Unspecified
W60.0 Conversion from previous arthrodesis and extraarticular bone graft nec

W61 Fusion of other joint and other articular bone graft

W61.1 Primary arthrodesis and articular bone graft nec
Includes: *Arthrodesis and articular bone graft nec*
W61.2 Revision of arthrodesis and articular bone graft nec
W61.3 Conversion to arthrodesis and articular bone graft nec
Note: *Use subsidiary conversion from code as necessary*
W61.8 Other specified
W61.9 Unspecified
W61.0 Conversion from previous arthrodesis and articular bone graft nec

W62   **Other primary fusion of other joint**
            Includes: Fusion of joint nec

W62.1   Primary arthrodesis and internal fixation of joint nec
W62.2   Primary arthrodesis and external fixation of joint nec
W62.8   Other specified
W62.9   Unspecified
            Includes: Primary arthrodesis nec
                    Simple arthrodesis nec
                    Arthrodesis nec

W63   **Revisional fusion of other joint**

W63.1   Revision of arthrodesis and internal fixation nec
W63.2   Revision of arthrodesis and external fixation nec
W63.8   Other specified
W63.9   Unspecified
            Includes: Revision of simple arthrodesis nec
                    Revision of arthrodesis nec

W64   **Conversion to fusion of other joint**

W64.1   Conversion to arthrodesis and internal fixation nec
W64.2   Conversion to arthrodesis and external fixation nec
W64.8   Other specified
W64.9   Unspecified
            Includes: Conversion to simple arthrodesis nec
                    Conversion to arthrodesis nec
W64.0   Conversion from previous arthrodesis nec

W65   **Primary open reduction of traumatic dislocation of joint**
            Excludes: Some similar operations for correction of congenital deformity (X19-X27)

W65.1   Primary open reduction of fracture dislocation of joint and skeletal traction hfq
            Includes: Open reduction of fracture dislocation of joint and skeletal traction hfq
W65.2   Primary open reduction of traumatic dislocation of joint and skeletal traction nec
            Includes: Open reduction of traumatic dislocation of joint and skeletal traction nec
W65.3   Primary open reduction of fracture dislocation of joint nec
            Includes: Open reduction of fracture dislocation of joint nec
W65.8   Other specified
W65.9   Unspecified
            Includes: Open reduction of traumatic dislocation of joint nec
                    Open reduction of dislocation of joint nec

W66   **Primary closed reduction of traumatic dislocation of joint**
            Excludes: Some similar operations for correction of congenital deformity (X19-X27)

W66.1   Primary closed reduction of fracture dislocation of joint and skeletal traction hfq
            Includes: Closed reduction of fracture dislocation of joint and skeletal traction hfq
W66.2   Primary closed reduction of traumatic dislocation of joint and skeletal traction nec
            Includes: Closed reduction of traumatic dislocation of joint and skeletal traction nec
                    Reduction of traumatic dislocation of joint and skeletal traction nec
                    Reduction of dislocation of joint and skeletal traction nec
W66.3   Primary manipulative closed reduction of fracture dislocation of joint nec
            Includes: Closed reduction of fracture dislocation of joint nec
                    Manipulative reduction of fracture dislocation of joint nec
W66.8   Other specified
W66.9   Unspecified
            Includes: Manipulative reduction of traumatic dislocation of joint nec
                    Manipulative reduction of dislocation of joint nec
                    Reduction of traumatic dislocation of joint nec
                    Reduction of dislocation of joint nec

W67   **Secondary reduction of traumatic dislocation of joint**
Excludes: Some similar operations for correction of congenital deformity (X19-X27)

W67.1   Secondary open reduction of fracture dislocation of joint and skeletal traction hfq
W67.2   Secondary open reduction of traumatic dislocation of joint and skeletal traction nec
Includes: Secondary open reduction of dislocation of joint and skeletal traction nec
W67.3   Secondary open reduction of fracture dislocation of joint nec
W67.4   Secondary open reduction of traumatic dislocation of joint nec
Includes: Secondary open reduction of dislocation of joint nec
W67.5   Remanipulation of fracture dislocation of joint
W67.6   Remanipulation of traumatic dislocation of joint
Includes: Remanipulation of dislocation of joint nec
W67.8   Other specified
W67.9   Unspecified

W68   **Primary reduction of injury to growth plate**

W68.1   Open reduction of injury to growth plate and internal fixation hfq
W68.2   Open reduction of injury to growth plate and traction hfq
W68.3   Open reduction of injury to growth plate nec
W68.4   Closed reduction of injury to growth plate and internal fixation hfq
W68.5   Closed reduction of injury to growth plate and traction hfq
W68.6   Closed reduction of injury to growth plate nec
W68.8   Other specified
W68.9   Unspecified

W69   **Open operations on synovial membrane of joint**

W69.1   Total synovectomy
W69.2   Subtotal synovectomy
W69.3   Partial synovectomy
Includes: Synovectomy nec
W69.4   Open biopsy of synovial membrane of joint
Includes: Open biopsy of lesion of synovial membrane of joint
Biopsy of synovial membrane of joint nec
Biopsy of lesion of synovial membrane of joint nec
W69.5   Open division of synovial plica
W69.8   Other specified
W69.9   Unspecified

W70   **Open operations on semilunar cartilage**
Includes: Operations on semilunar cartilage nec

W70.1   Open total excision of semilunar cartilage
W70.2   Open excision of semilunar cartilage nec
Includes: Open excision of lesion of semilunar cartilage
W70.3   Open repair of semilunar cartilage
W70.8   Other specified
W70.9   Unspecified

W71   **Other open operations on intraarticular structure**
Includes: Operations on intraarticular structure nec

W71.1   Open drilling of articular cartilage
W71.2   Open excision of intraarticular osteophyte
W71.3   Forage of joint
W71.8   Other specified
W71.9   Unspecified

W72 Prosthetic replacement of ligament

W72.1 Primary prosthetic replacement of multiple ligaments
W72.2 Prosthetic replacement of multiple ligaments nec
W72.3 Primary prosthetic replacement of intraarticular ligament
W72.4 Prosthetic replacement of intraarticular ligament nec
W72.5 Primary prosthetic replacement of extraarticular ligament
W72.6 Prosthetic replacement of extraarticular ligament nec
W72.8 Other specified
W72.9 Unspecified

W73 Prosthetic reinforcement of ligament

W73.1 Primary extraarticular prosthetic augmentation of intraarticular ligament nec
W73.2 Extraarticular prosthetic augmentation of intraarticular ligament nec
W73.3 Primary prosthetic reinforcement of intraarticular ligament nec
W73.4 Prosthetic reinforcement of intraarticular ligament nec
W73.8 Other specified
W73.9 Unspecified

W74 Other reconstruction of ligament

W74.1 Reconstruction of multiple ligaments nec
W74.2 Reconstruction of intraarticular ligament nec
W74.3 Reconstruction of extraarticular ligament nec
W74.8 Other specified
W74.9 Unspecified

W75 Other open repair of ligament
Includes: Repair of ligament nec

W75.1 Open repair of multiple ligaments nec
W75.2 Open repair of intraarticular ligament nec
W75.3 Open repair of extraarticular ligament nec
W75.8 Other specified
W75.9 Unspecified

W76 Other operations on ligament

W76.1 Excision of ligament
W76.2 Excision of lesion of ligament
W76.3 Biopsy of lesion of ligament
Includes: Biopsy of ligamet
W76.8 Other specified
W76.9 Unspecified

W77 Stabilising operations on joint
Excludes: Some similar operations for correction of congenital deformity (X19-X27)

W77.1 Repair of capsule of joint for stabilisation of joint
W77.2 Transposition of muscle for stabilisation of joint
W77.3 Blocking operations on joint using prosthesis for stabilisation of joint
W77.4 Blocking operations on joint using bone for stabilisation of joint
W77.5 Periarticular osteotomy for stabilisation of joint
W77.8 Other specified
W77.9 Unspecified

W78 Release of contracture of joint
Excludes: Some similar operations for correction of congenital deformity (X19-X27)

W78.1 Release of contracture of shoulder joint
W78.2 Release of contracture of hip joint
W78.3 Release of contracture of knee joint
W78.4 Limited release of contracture of capsule of joint
W78.8 Other specified
W78.9 Unspecified

W79   Soft tissue operations on joint of toe
         Excludes: Some similar operations for correction of congenital deformity (X19-X27)

W79.1   Soft tissue correction of hallux valgus
         Include: Soft tissue correction of hallux valgus and excision of bunion
         Note: Use supplementary code for concurrent osteotomy of first metatarsal bone (W15)
                     Use supplementary code for concurrent arthrodesis (W60)
W79.2   Excision of bunion nec
         Includes: Bunionectomy
                   Simple excision of bunion
                   Excision of bunionette
W79.3   Syndactylisation of lesser toes
W79.8   Other specified
W79.9   Unspecified

W81   Other open operations on joint
         Excludes: Some similar operations for correction of congenital deformity (X19-X27)

W81.1   Excision of lesion of joint nec
W81.2   Open removal of loose body from joint
W81.3   Drainage of joint
W81.4   Incision of joint nec
         Includes: Arthrotomy nec
W81.5   Exploration of joint nec
W81.8   Other specified
W81.9   Unspecified

W82   Therapeutic endoscopic operations on semilunar cartilage
         Note: It is not necessary to code additionally any mention of diagnostic endoscopic examination of
                     knee joint (W87.9)

W82.1   Endoscopic total excision of semilunar cartilage
W82.2   Endoscopic resection of semilunar cartilage nec
W82.3   Endoscopic repair of semilunar cartilage
W82.8   Other specified
W82.9   Unspecified

W83   Therapeutic endoscopic operations on other articular cartilage
         Note: It is not necessary to code additionally any mention of diagnostic endoscopic examination of
                     same joint (W87.9 W88.9)

W83.1   Endoscopic drilling of lesion of articular cartilage
W83.2   Endoscopic fixation of lesion of articular cartilage
W83.3   Endoscopic shaving of articular cartilage
W83.8   Other specified
W83.9   Unspecified

W84   Therapeutic endoscopic operations on other joint structure
         Note: It is not necessary to code additionally any mention of diagnostic endoscopic examination of
                     same joint (W87.9 W88.9)

W84.1   Endoscopic repair of intraarticular ligament
W84.2   Endoscopic reattachment of intraarticular ligament
W84.3   Endoscopic division of synovial plica
W84.8   Other specified
W84.9   Unspecified

W85   Therapeutic endoscopic operations on cavity of knee joint
         Note: It is not necessary to code additionally any mention of diagnostic endoscopic examination of
                     knee joint (W87.9)

W85.1   Endoscopic removal of loose body from knee joint
W85.2   Endoscopic irrigation of knee joint
         Includes: Endoscopic lavage of knee joint
                   Endoscopic washout of knee joint
W85.8   Other specified
W85.9   Unspecified

W86 **Therapeutic endoscopic operations on cavity of other joint**
Note: *It is not necessary to code additionally any mention of diagnostic endoscopic examination of same joint (W88.9)*

W86.1   Endoscopic removal of loose body from joint nec
W86.8   Other specified
W86.9   Unspecified

W87 **Diagnostic endoscopic examination of knee joint**

W87.1   Diagnostic endoscopic examination of knee joint and biopsy of lesion of knee joint
        Includes: Diagnostic endoscopic examination of knee joint and biopsy of knee joint
                 Endoscopic biopsy of lesion of knee joint
                 Endoscopic biopsy of knee joint
W87.8   Other specified
W87.9   Unspecified
        Includes: Arthroscopy of knee joint nec

W88 **Diagnostic endoscopic examination of other joint**

W88.1   Diagnostic endoscopic examination of joint and biopsy of lesion of joint nec
        Includes: Diagnostic endoscopic examination of joint and biopsy of joint nec
                 Endoscopic biopsy of lesion of joint nec
                 Endoscopic biopsy of joint nec
W88.8   Other specified
W88.9   Unspecified
        Includes: Arthroscopy nec

W90 **Puncture of joint**

W90.1   Aspiration of joint
W90.2   Arthrography
W90.3   Injection of therapeutic substance into joint
W90.4   Injection into joint nec
W90.8   Other specified
W90.9   Unspecified

W91 **Other manipulation of joint**

W91.1   Manipulation of joint using traction nec
W91.8   Other specified
W91.9   Unspecified

W92 **Other operations on joint**
        Excludes: Some similar operations for correction of congenital deformity (X19-X27)

W92.1   Biopsy of lesion of joint nec
        Includes: Biopsy of joint nec
W92.2   Distension of joint
W92.3   Examination of joint under image intensifier
W92.4   Examination of joint under anaesthetic
W92.5   Examination of joint nec
W92.8   Other specified
W92.9   Unspecified

CHAPTER X

MISCELLANEOUS OPERATIONS

(CODES X01-X59)

Includes: OPERATIONS COVERING MULTIPLE SYSTEMS

Note: *This chapter contains certain codes designed to precede codes in Chapter Y when more precise preceding codes cannot be determined or are not applicable*

X01   Replantation of upper limb

X01.1   Replantation of whole arm
X01.2   Replantation of forearm
X01.3   Replantation of hand
X01.4   Replantation of thumb
X01.5   Replantation of finger nec
X01.8   Other specified
X01.9   Unspecified
         Includes: Replantation of arm nec

X02   Replantation of lower limb

X02.1   Replantation of whole leg
X02.2   Replantation of foot
X02.3   Replantation of toe
X02.8   Other specified
X02.9   Unspecified
         Includes: Replantation of leg nec

X03   Replantation of other organ

X03.1   Replantation of ear
X03.2   Replantation of nose
X03.8   Other specified
X03.9   Unspecified

X04   Transplantation between systems

X04.1   Autotransplantation of adrenal medulla to caudate nucleus of brain
X04.8   Other specified
X04.9   Unspecified

X05   Implantation of prosthesis for limb

X05.1   Implantation of bioelectrical prosthesis for limb
X05.2   Implantation of kineplastic prosthesis for limb
X05.3   Attention to prosthesis for limb
X05.8   Other specified
X05.9   Unspecified

X07   Amputation of arm

X07.1   Forequarter amputation
X07.2   Disarticulation of shoulder
X07.3   Amputation of arm above elbow
X07.4   Amputation of arm through elbow
X07.5   Amputation of arm through forearm
X07.8   Other specified
X07.9   Unspecified

X08 Amputation of hand

X08.1 Amputation of hand at wrist
X08.2 Amputation of thumb
 Excludes: Amputation of duplicate thumb (X21.5)
X08.3 Amputation of phalanx of finger
X08.4 Amputation of finger nec
 Excludes: Amputation of supernumerary finger (X21.6)
X08.8 Other specified
X08.9 Unspecified

X09 Amputation of leg

X09.1 Hindquarter amputation
X09.2 Disarticulation of hip
X09.3 Amputation of leg above knee
X09.4 Amputation of leg through knee
X09.5 Amputation of leg below knee
X09.8 Other specified
X09.9 Unspecified

X10 Amputation of foot

X10.1 Amputation of foot through ankle
X10.2 Disarticulation of tarsal bones
X10.3 Disarticulation of metatarsal bones
X10.4 Amputation through metatarsal bones
X10.8 Other specified
X10.9 Unspecified

X11 Amputation of toe
Excludes: Amputation of supernumerary toe (X27.3)

X11.1 Amputation of great toe
X11.2 Amputation of phalanx of toe
X11.8 Other specified
X11.9 Unspecified
 Includes: Disarticulation of toe

X12 Operations on amputation stump

X12.1 Reamputation at higher level
X12.2 Excision of lesion of amputation stump
X12.3 Shortening of length of amputation stump
X12.4 Revision of coverage of amputation stump
X12.5 Drainage of amputation stump
X12.8 Other specified
X12.9 Unspecified

X14 Clearance of pelvis

X14.1 Total exenteration of pelvis
 Includes: Exenteration of pelvis nec
X14.2 Anterior exenteration of pelvis
X14.3 Posterior exenteration of pelvis
X14.8 Other specified
X14.9 Unspecified

X15 Operations for sexual transformation

X15.1 Combined operations for transformation from male to female
X15.2 Combined operations for transformation from female to male
X15.3 Excision of ovotestis
X15.8 Other specified
X15.9 Unspecified

X17   **Separation of conjoined twins**

X17.1   Combined operations to separate conjoined twins
X17.8   Other specified
X17.9   Unspecified

X19   **Correction of congenital deformity of shoulder or upper arm**

X19.1   Reduction of sprengel deformity
X19.2   Correction of obstetric palsy
X19.8   Other specified
X19.9   Unspecified

X20   **Correction of congenital deformity of forearm**

X20.1   Excision of anlage of radius
X20.2   Excision of anlage of ulna
X20.3   Centralisation of carpus for correction of congenital deformity of forearm
X20.4   Revision of release of radius for correction of congenital deformity of forearm
X20.5   Revision of release of ulna for correction of congenital deformity of forearm
X20.8   Other specified
X20.9   Unspecified

X21   **Correction of congenital deformity of hand**

X21.1   Reduction of gigantism of hand
X21.2   Correction of mirror hand
X21.3   Correction of syndactyly of fingers using skin graft
X21.4   Correction of syndactyly of fingers using skin expander
X21.5   Amputation of duplicate thumb
X21.6   Amputation of supernumerary finger nec
X21.8   Other specified
X21.9   Unspecified

X22   **Correction of congenital deformity of hip**

X22.1   Open reduction of congenital deformity of hip
X22.2   Primary osteotomy of pelvis for correction of congenital deformity of hip
         Includes: Osteotomy of pelvis for correction of congenital deformity of hip
X22.3   Secondary arthroplasty of hip for correction of congenital deformity of hip
X22.4   Intraarticular soft tissue procedures for correction of congenital deformity of hip
X22.5   Extraarticular procedures for correction of congenital deformity of hip
X22.8   Other specified
X22.9   Unspecified

X23   **Correction of congenital deformity of leg**

X23.1   Operative reduction of congenital dislocation of knee
X23.2   Correction of pseudarthrosis of tibia
X23.3   Excision of anlage of fibula
X23.4   Excision of anlage of tibia
X23.5   Centralisation of tarsus for correction of congenital deformity of leg
X23.6   Reversal of rotation plasty of ankle for correction of congenital deformity of leg
X23.8   Other specified
X23.9   Unspecified

X24   **Primary correction of congenital deformity of foot**

X24.1   Release of pantalar joints for correction of congenital deformity of foot
X24.2   Posterior release of joints of foot for correction of congenital deformity of foot
X24.3   Medial release of joints of foot for correction of congenital deformity of foot
X24.4   Anterior release of joints of foot for correction of congenital deformity of foot
X24.8   Other specified
X24.9   Unspecified

X25 Other correction of congenital deformity of foot
Includes: Late correction of congenital deformity of foot

X25.1 Osteotomy of body of os calcis
X25.2 Wedge tarsectomy for correction of congenital deformity of foot
X25.3 Reduction of gigantism of foot
X25.4 Separation of tarsal coalition
X25.8 Other specified
X25.9 Unspecified

X27 Correction of minor congenital deformity of foot

X27.1 Release of streeter band
X27.2 Release of syndactyly of toes
X27.3 Amputation of supernumerary toe
X27.4 Correction of curly fifth toe
X27.5 Correction of congenital crossed toes
X27.8 Other specified
X27.9 Unspecified

X29 Continuous infusion of therapeutic substance

X29.1 Continuous subcutaneous infusion of insulin
X29.8 Other specified
X29.9 Unspecified

X30 Injection of therapeutic substance
Includes: Injection of prophylactic substance

X30.1 Injection of rh immune globulin
X30.2 Injection of gamma globulin
X30.3 Injection of immune serum nec
X30.8 Other specified
X30.9 Unspecified

X31 Injection of radiocontrast material

X31.1 Intravenous cholecystography
X31.2 Intravenous pyelography
X31.3 Intravenous injection of radiocontrast material nec
X31.8 Other specified
X31.9 Unspecified

X32 Exchange blood transfusion

X32.1 Neonatal exchange blood transfusion
X32.8 Other specified
X32.9 Unspecified

X33 Other blood transfusion

X33.1 Intraarterial blood transfusion
X33.2 Intravenous blood transfusion of packed cells
X33.3 Intravenous blood transfusion of platelets
X33.8 Other specified
X33.9 Unspecified
Includes: Intravenous blood transfusion nec

X34 Other intravenous transfusion

X34.1 Transfusion of coagulation factor
X34.2 Transfusion of plasma
X34.3 Transfusion of serum nec
X34.4 Transfusion of blood expander
X34.8 Other specified
X34.9 Unspecified

X35 Other intravenous injection

X35.1 Intravenous induction of labour
X35.2 Intravenous chemotherapy
X35.3 Intravenous immunotherapy
X35.4 Intravenous injection of non radioactive diagnostic substance
X35.8 Other specified
X35.9 Unspecified

X36 Blood withdrawal

X36.1 Blood donation
X36.2 Venesection
X36.8 Other specified
X36.9 Unspecified

X37 Intramuscular injection

X37.1 Intramuscular calcitonin therapy
X37.2 Intramuscular gold therapy
X37.3 Intramuscular chemotherapy
X37.4 Intramuscular immunotherapy
X37.5 Intramuscular injection for local action
X37.8 Other specified
X37.9 Unspecified

X38 Subcutaneous injection

X38.1 Injection of triamcinolone for local action
X38.2 Injection of steroid for local action nec
X38.3 Injection of hormone for local action nec
X38.4 Subcutaneous chemotherapy
X38.5 Subcutaneous immunotherapy
X38.6 Subcutaneous injection for local action nec
X38.8 Other specified
X38.9 Unspecified

X40 Compensation for renal failure

X40.1 Renal dialysis
X40.2 Peritoneal dialysis
X40.3 Haemodialysis nec
X40.8 Other specified
X40.9 Unspecified

X41 Placement of ambulatory apparatus for compensation for renal failure

X41.1 Insertion of ambulatory peritoneal dialysis catheter
X41.2 Removal of ambulatory peritoneal dialysis catheter
X41.8 Other specified
X41.9 Unspecified

X42 Placement of other apparatus for compensation for renal failure

X42.1 Insertion of temporary peritoneal dialysis catheter
X42.8 Other specified
X42.9 Unspecified

X45 Donation of organ

X45.1 Donation of kidney
X45.8 Other specified
X45.9 Unspecified

X46   **Donation of other tissue**

X46.1   Donation of bone marrow
X46.2   Donation of skin
X46.8   Other specified
X46.9   Unspecified

X48   **Immobilisation using plaster cast**

X48.1   Application of plaster cast
         Note: *This code is not normally used when associated with another operation for treatment of fracture or disease of bone (Chapter V-W)*
X48.2   Change of plaster cast
X48.3   Removal of plaster cast
X48.8   Other specified
X48.9   Unspecified

X49   **Other immobilisation**
         Note: *These codes are not normally used when associated with another operation for treatment of fracture or disease of bone (Chapter V-W)*

X49.1   Application of splint nec
X49.2   Change of splint nec
X49.3   Removal of splint nec
X49.4   Skin traction
X49.8   Other specified
X49.9   Unspecified

X50   **External resuscitation**

X50.1   Direct current cardioversion
X50.2   External cardioversion nec
X50.8   Other specified
X50.9   Unspecified

X51   **Change of body temperature**

X51.1   Hypothermia therapy
X51.8   Other specified
X51.9   Unspecified

X53   **Extirpation of unspecified organ**

X53.1   Excision of unspecified organ
X53.2   Excision of lesion of unspecified organ
X53.3   Destruction of lesion of unspecified organ
X53.8   Other specified
X53.9   Unspecified

X55   **Other operations on unspecified organ**

X55.1   Biopsy of lesion of unspecified organ
         Includes: Biopsy of unspecified organ
X55.2   Incision of unspecified organ
X55.8   Other specified
X55.9   Unspecified

X59   **Anaesthetic without surgery**

X59.1   Preoperative anaesthetic death
X59.8   Other specified
X59.9   Unspecified

CHAPTER Y

SUBSIDIARY CLASSIFICATION OF
METHODS OF OPERATION

(CODES Y01-Y90)

Includes: OPERATIONS WITHOUT SPECIFIC SITE ANAESTHETIC METHODS

Excludes: ANAESTHETIC WITHOUT SURGERY   (Chapter X)

Note: Codes in this chapter are not intended as primary codes

Y01   Replacement of organ noc

Y01.1   Autoreplacement of organ noc
Y01.2   Alloreplacement of organ noc
Y01.3   Xenoreplacement of organ noc
Y01.8   Other specified
Y01.9   Unspecified

Y02   Placement of prosthesis in organ noc

Y02.1   Implantation of prosthesis into organ noc
Y02.2   Insertion of prosthesis into organ noc
Y02.8   Other specified
Y02.9   Unspecified

Y03   Attention to prosthesis in organ noc

Y03.1   Maintenance of prosthesis in organ noc
Y03.2   Renewal of prosthesis in organ noc
Y03.3   Correction of displacement of prosthesis noc
Y03.4   Other resiting of prosthesis in organ noc
Y03.5   Conversion to prosthesis in organ noc
Y03.6   Adjustment to prosthesis in organ noc
Y03.7   Removal of prosthesis from organ noc
Y03.8   Other specified
Y03.9   Unspecified

Y04   Replantation of organ noc

Y04.1   Microvascular reattachment of organ noc
Y04.8   Other specified
Y04.9   Unspecified

Y05   Excision of organ noc

Y05.1   Total excision of organ noc
Y05.2   Partial excision of organ noc
Y05.3   Excision of sinus track from organ noc
         Includes: Excision of fistula from organ noc
         Note: Site specific chapter related code can be used only when precise identification of organ
                     from which sinus track or fistula originates is given
                     This does not include skin of site of original operation
                     Otherwise X55.8 should be used
Y05.8   Other specified
Y05.9   Unspecified

Y06 **Excision of lesion of organ noc**

Y06.1 Marsupialisation of organ noc
Y06.2 Deroofing of cyst of organ noc
Y06.3 Enucleation of lesion of organ noc
Y06.4 Excision of scar tissue noc
Y06.8 Other specified
Y06.9 Unspecified

Y07 **Obliteration of cavity of organ noc**

Y07.1 Ligation of organ noc
Y07.2 Clipping of organ noc
Y07.3 Obliteration of sinus track from organ noc
Includes: Obliteration of fistula from organ noc
Closure of sinus track from organ noc
Closure of fistula from organ noc
Note: *Site specific chapter related code can be used only when precise identification of organ*
from which sinus track or fistula originates is given
This does not include skin of site of original operation
Otherwise X55.8 should be used
Y07.4 Obliteration of diverticulum of organ noc
Y07.8 Other specified
Y07.9 Unspecified

Y08 **Laser therapy to organ noc**

Y08.1 Laser excision of organ noc
Y08.2 Laser excision of lesion of organ noc
Y08.3 Laser destruction of organ noc
Y08.4 Laser destruction of lesion of organ noc
Y08.8 Other specified
Y08.9 Unspecified

Y09 **Chemical destruction of organ noc**

Y09.1 Injection of sclerosing substance into organ noc
Includes: Sclerotherapy to organ noc
Y09.2 Injection of other destructive substance into organ noc
Y09.8 Other specified
Y09.9 Unspecified

Y11 **Other destruction of organ noc**

Y11.1 Cauterisation of organ noc
Y11.2 Cryotherapy to organ noc
Y11.3 Curettage of organ noc
Y11.4 Radiofrequency controlled thermal destruction of organ noc
Y11.5 Ultrasonic destruction of organ noc
Y11.8 Other specified
Y11.9 Unspecified

Y12 **Chemical destruction of lesion of organ noc**

Y12.1 Injection of sclerosing substance into lesion of organ noc
Includes: Sclerotherapy to lesion of organ noc
Y12.2 Injection of other destructive substance into lesion of organ noc
Y12.8 Other specified
Y12.9 Unspecified

Y13   **Other destruction of lesion of organ noc**

Y13.1   Cauterisation of lesion of organ noc
Y13.2   Cryotherapy to lesion of organ noc
Y13.3   Curettage of lesion of organ noc
Y13.4   Radiofrequency controlled thermal destruction of lesion of organ noc
Y13.5   Ultrasonic destruction of lesion of organ noc
Y13.8   Other specified
Y13.9   Unspecified

Y16   **Connection of organ noc**

Y16.1   Exteriorisation of organ noc
Y16.2   Anastomosis of organ noc
Y16.3   Bypass of organ noc
Y16.8   Other specified
Y16.9   Unspecified

Y18   **Release of organ noc**

Y18.1   Freeing of adhesions of organ noc
Y18.8   Other specified
Y18.9   Unspecified

Y20   **Biopsy of organ noc**

Y20.1   Stereotactic biopsy of lesion of organ noc
Y20.2   Stereotactic biopsy of organ noc
Y20.3   Biopsy of lesion of organ noc
Y20.8   Other specified
Y20.9   Unspecified

Y21   **Cytology of organ noc**

Y21.1   Brush cytology of organ noc
Y21.8   Other specified
Y21.9   Unspecified

Y22   **Drainage of organ noc**

Y22.1   Aspiration of haematoma of organ noc
Y22.2   Aspiration of other lesion of organ noc
Y22.3   Irrigation of organ noc
        Includes: Lavage of organ noc
        *   Washout of organ noc*
Y22.8   Other specified
Y22.9   Unspecified

Y24   **Microvascular repair of organ noc**

Y24.1   Microvascular reconstruction of organ noc
Y24.2   Attention to microvascular repair of organ noc
Y24.8   Other specified
Y24.9   Unspecified

Y25   **Suture of organ noc**

Y25.1   Suture of laceration of organ noc
Y25.2   Resuture of organ noc
Y25.3   Removal of retained suture from organ noc
Y25.4   Removal of other suture from organ noc
Y25.5   Other attention to suture of organ noc
Y25.8   Other specified
Y25.9   Unspecified

Y26   Other repair of organ noc

Y26.1   Reconstruction of organ noc
Y26.2   Plastic repair of organ noc
Y26.3   Stapling of organ noc
Y26.4   Removal of other repair material from organ noc
Y26.5   Other attention to repair of organ noc
Y26.8   Other specified
Y26.9   Unspecified

Y27   Graft to organ noc

Y27.1   Autograft to organ noc
Y27.2   Allograft to organ noc
Y27.3   Xenograft to organ noc
Y27.4   Attention to graft of organ noc
Y27.8   Other specified
Y27.9   Unspecified

Y29   Removal of foreign body from organ noc

Y29.1   Surgical removal of foreign body from organ noc
Y29.2   Manipulative removal of foreign body from organ noc
Y29.8   Other specified
Y29.9   Unspecified

Y30   Incision of organ noc

Y30.1   Incision of lesion of organ noc
Y30.8   Other specified
Y30.9   Unspecified

Y31   Exploration of organ noc

Y31.1   Exploration of sinus track from organ noc
         Includes: Exploration of fistula from organ noc
         Note: Site specific chapter related code can be used only when precise identification of organ
         *   from which sinus track or fistula originates is given*
         *   This does not include skin of site of original operation*
         *   Otherwise X55.8 should be used*
Y31.8   Other specified
Y31.9   Unspecified

Y32   Reexploration of organ noc

Y32.1   Reexploration of organ and surgical arrest of postoperative bleeding noc
Y32.2   Reexploration of organ and other repair of organ noc
         Includes: Reexploration of organ and resuture of organ noc
Y32.3   Reexploration of organ and packing of organ noc
Y32.8   Other specified
Y32.9   Unspecified

Y33   Puncture of organ noc

Y33.1   Acupuncture of organ noc
Y33.2   Drilling of organ noc
Y33.8   Other specified
Y33.9   Unspecified

Y35   Introduction of removable radioactive material into organ noc

Y35.1   Introduction of radioactive caesium into organ noc
Y35.2   Introduction of iridium wire into organ noc
Y35.3   Introduction of radium into organ noc
Y35.8   Other specified
Y35.9   Unspecified

Y36　　**Introduction of non removable material into organ noc**

Y36.1　Introduction of gold seeds into organ noc
Y36.2　Introduction of therapeutic implant into organ noc
Y36.8　Other specified
Y36.9　Unspecified

Y38　　**Injection of therapeutic inclusion substance into organ noc**

Y38.1　Continuous injection of therapeutic substance into organ noc
Y38.8　Other specified
Y38.9　Unspecified

Y39　　**Injection of other substance into organ noc**

Y39.1　Injection of radiocontrast substance into sinus track from organ noc
　　　Includes: Injection of radiocontrast substance into fistula from organ noc
　　　　　　Sinogram noc
　　　Note:　Site specific chapter related code can be used only when precise identification of organ
　　　　　from which sinus track or fistula originates is given
　　　　　This does not include skin of site of original operation
　　　　　Otherwise X55.8 should be used
Y39.2　Other injection of radiocontrast substance into organ noc
Y39.3　Injection of inert substance into organ noc
Y39.8　Other specified
Y39.9　Unspecified

Y40　　**Dilation of organ noc**

Y40.1　Dilation of stricture of organ noc
Y40.2　Stretching of organ noc
Y40.8　Other specified
Y40.9　Unspecified

Y41　　**Examination of organ noc**

Y41.1　Examination of organ under anaesthetic noc
Y41.8　Other specified
Y41.9　Unspecified

Y42　　**Manipulation of organ noc**

Y42.1　External manipulation of organ noc
Y42.8　Other specified
Y42.9　Unspecified

Y44　　**Other methods of operation on organ noc**

Y44.1　Evacuation of contents of organ noc
Y44.2　Monitoring of pressure in organ noc
Y44.8　Other specified
Y44.9　Unspecified

Y46　　**Open approach to contents of cranium**

Y46.1　Transsphenoidal open approach to contents of cranium
Y46.2　Frontal open approach to contents of cranium
Y46.3　Transoral open approach to contents of cranium
Y46.4　Transmastoid open approach to contents of cranium
Y46.5　Supratentorial open approach to contents of cranium
Y46.6　Infratentorial open approach to contents of cranium
Y46.8　Other specified
Y46.9　Unspecified

Y47 **Burrhole approach to contents of cranium**

Y47.1   Transsphenoidal burrhole approach to contents of cranium
Y47.2   Frontal burrhole approach to contents of cranium
Y47.3   Transoral burrhole approach to contents of cranium
Y47.4   Transmastoid burrhole approach to contents of cranium
Y47.5   Supratentorial burrhole approach to contents of cranium
Y47.6   Infratentorial burrhole approach to contents of cranium
Y47.8   Other specified
Y47.9   Unspecified

Y48 **Approach to spine through back**

Y48.1   Laminectomy approach to cervical spine
Y48.2   Laminectomy approach to thoracic spine
Y48.3   Laminectomy approach to lumbar spine
Y48.8   Other specified
Y48.9   Unspecified
        Includes: Laminectomy approach to spine nec

Y49 **Approach through thoracic cavity**

Y49.1   Median sternotomy approach
Y49.2   Transthoracic approach to spine
Y49.3   Thoracotomy approach nec
Y49.8   Other specified
Y49.9   Unspecified

Y50 **Approach through abdominal cavity**

Y50.1   Transperitoneal approach to spine
Y50.2   Laparotomy approach nec
Y50.3   Vaginal approach
Y50.8   Other specified
Y50.9   Unspecified

Y51 **Approach to organ through artificial opening into gastrointestinal tract**

Y51.1   Approach to organ through oesophagostomy
Y51.2   Approach to organ through gastrostomy
Y51.3   Approach to organ through ileostomy
Y51.4   Approach to organ through colostomy
Y51.8   Other specified
Y51.9   Unspecified

Y52 **Approach to organ through other artificial opening**

Y52.1   Approach to organ through tracheostomy
Y52.2   Approach to organ through urethrostomy
Y52.3   Approach to organ through cystostomy
Y52.8   Other specified
Y52.9   Unspecified

Y53 **Percutaneous approach to organ under image control**

Y53.1   Percutaneous approach to organ under radiological control
Y53.2   Percutaneous approach to organ under ultrasonic control
Y53.3   Percutaneous approach to organ under cat scan control
Y53.8   Other specified
Y53.9   Unspecified

Y54 **Harvest of nerve**

Y54.1 Harvest of sural nerve
Y54.2 Harvest of nerve of head
  Includes: Harvest of nerve of neck
Y54.3 Harvest of peripheral nerve nec
Y54.8 Other specified
Y54.9 Unspecified

Y55 **Harvest of random pattern flap of skin from limb**

Y55.1 Harvest of random pattern flap of skin from hand
Y55.2 Harvest of random pattern flap of skin from upper arm
Y55.3 Harvest of random pattern flap of skin from arm nec
Y55.4 Harvest of random pattern flap of skin from foot
Y55.5 Harvest of random pattern flap of skin from thigh
Y55.6 Harvest of random pattern flap of skin from leg nec
Y55.8 Other specified
Y55.9 Unspecified

Y56 **Harvest of random pattern·flap of skin from other site**

Y56.1 Harvest of random pattern flap of skin from head
  Includes: Harvest of random pattern flap of skin from neck
Y56.2 Harvest of random pattern flap of skin from back
Y56.3 Harvest of random pattern flap of skin from chest
Y56.4 Harvest of random pattern flap of skin from abdomen
Y56.8 Other specified
Y56.9 Unspecified

Y57 **Harvest of axial pattern flap of skin**

Y57.1 Harvest of axial pattern flap of skin from forehead
Y57.2 Harvest of axial pattern cross lip flap of skin
Y57.3 Harvest of axial pattern flap of skin from scapular region
Y57.4 Harvest of axial pattern flap of skin from deltopectoral region
Y57.5 Harvest of axial pattern flap of skin from inferior epigastric region
Y57.6 Harvest of axial pattern flap of skin from groin
Y57.8 Other specified
Y57.9 Unspecified

Y58 **Harvest of skin for graft**

Y58.1 Harvest of full thickness skin from post auricular region
Y58.8 Other specified
Y58.9 Unspecified

Y59 **Harvest of flap of skin and fascia**

Y59.1 Harvest of temporalis flap of skin and fascia
Y59.2 Harvest of radial artery flap of skin and fascia
Y59.3 Harvest of ulna artery flap of skin and fascia
Y59.4 Harvest of lateral arm flap of skin and fascia
Y59.5 Harvest of posterior interosseous flap of skin and fascia
Y59.6 Harvest of lower leg flap of skin and fascia
Y59.8 Other specified
Y59.9 Unspecified

Y60 **Other harvest of fascia**

Y60.1 Harvest of sheet of fascia from fascia lata
Y60.2 Harvest of fascia from fascia lata nec
Y60.3 Harvest of sheet of fascia from abdominal wall
Y60.4 Harvest of fascia from abdominal wall nec
Y60.5 Harvest of sheet of fascia from pleural cavity
Y60.8 Other specified
Y60.9 Unspecified

Y61   Harvest of flap of skin and muscle of trunk

Y61.1   Harvest of flap of skin and trapezius muscle
Y61.2   Harvest of flap of skin and pectoralis major muscle
Y61.3   Harvest of flap of skin and latissimus dorsi muscle
Y61.4   Harvest of flap of skin and gluteus maximus muscle
Y61.5   Harvest of flap of skin and rectus abdominis muscle
Y61.8   Other specified
Y61.9   Unspecified

Y62   Harvest of flap of skin and muscle of other site

Y62.1   Harvest of flap of skin and sternomastoid muscle
Y62.2   Harvest of flap of skin and tensor fasciae latae muscle
Y62.3   Harvest of flap of skin and gastrocnemius muscle
Y62.8   Other specified
Y62.9   Unspecified

Y63   Harvest of flap of muscle of trunk

Y63.1   Harvest of flap of latissimus dorsi muscle nec
Y63.2   Harvest of flap of serratus anterior muscle
Y63.3   Harvest of flap of inferior epigastric muscle
Y63.8   Other specified
Y63.9   Unspecified

Y64   Harvest of flap of muscle of other site

Y64.1   Harvest of flap of temporalis muscle
Y64.2   Harvest of flap of gracilis muscle
Y64.3   Harvest of flap of gastrocnemius muscle nec
Y64.4   Harvest of flap of soleus muscle
Y64.5   Harvest of flap of extensor digitorum brevis muscle
Y64.8   Other specified
Y64.9   Unspecified

Y65   Harvest of tendon

Y65.1   Harvest of palmaris longus tendon
Y65.2   Harvest of plantaris tendon
Y65.3   Harvest of extensor tendon of toe
Y65.8   Other specified
Y65.9   Unspecified

Y66   Harvest of bone

Y66.1   Harvest of bone from skull
Y66.2   Harvest of bone from rib
Y66.3   Harvest of bone from iliac crest
Y66.4   Harvest of bone from radius
Y66.5   Harvest of bone from ulna
Y66.6   Harvest of bone from fibula
Y66.7   Harvest of bone marrow
Y66.8   Other specified
Y66.9   Unspecified

Y67   Harvest of other multiple tissue

Y67.1   Harvest of composite of skin and cartilage from ear
Y67.8   Other specified
Y67.9   Unspecified

Y69   **Harvest of other tissue**

Y69.1   Harvest of omentum
Y69.8   Other specified
Y69.9   Unspecified

Y70   **Early operations noc**

Y70.1   Emergency operations noc
Y70.2   Immediate operations noc
Y70.3   First stage of staged operations noc
Y70.4   Primary operations noc
Y70.5   Temporary operations
Y70.8   Other specified
Y70.9   Unspecified

Y71   **Late operations noc**

Y71.1   Subsequent stage of staged operations noc
Y71.2   Secondary operations noc
Y71.3   Revisional operations noc
Y71.8   Other specified
Y71.9   Unspecified

Y73   **Facilitating operations noc**

Y73.1   Cardiopulmonary bypass
Y73.2   Extracorporeal circulation nec
Y73.8   Other specified
Y73.9   Unspecified

ANAESTHETICS

These do not qualify as operations or procedures as defined on pages ix and x of the Introduction. Therefore these codes should not be used to identify such

Y80   **General anaesthetic**

Y80.1   Inhalation anaesthetic using muscle relaxant
Y80.2   Inhalation anaesthetic using endotracheal intubation nec
Y80.3   Inhalation anaesthetic nec
Y80.4   Intravenous anaesthetic nec
Y80.8   Other specified
Y80.9   Unspecified

Y81   **Spinal anaesthetic**

Y81.1   Epidural anaesthetic using lumbar approach
          Includes: Epidural anaesthetic nec
Y81.2   Epidural anaesthetic using sacral approach
Y81.8   Other specified
Y81.9   Unspecified

Y82   **Local anaesthetic**

Y82.1   Local anaesthetic nerve block
          Excludes: Destructive nerve block (Chapter A)
Y82.2   Injection of local anaesthetic nec
Y82.3   Application of local anaesthetic
Y82.8   Other specified
Y82.9   Unspecified

Y84   Other anaesthetic

Y84.1   Gas and air analgesia in labour
Y84.8   Other specified
Y84.9   Unspecified

NONOPERATIONS

These do not qualify as operations or procedures as defined on pages ix and x of the Introduction. Therefore these codes should not be used to identify such

Y90   Other nonoperations

Y90.1   Application of transcutaneous electrical nerve stimulator
Y90.2   Radiotherapy nec
Y90.3   Scanning nec
Y90.4   Barium meal
Y90.5   Barium enema nec
Y90.8   Other specified
Y90.9   Unspecified

CHAPTER Z

SUBSIDIARY CLASSIFICATION OF SITES OF OPERATION

(CODES Z01-Z94)

Note: Codes in this chapter are not intended as primary codes

Z01   **Tissue of brain**

Z01.1   Tissue of frontal lobe of brain
Z01.2   Tissue of temporal lobe of brain
Z01.3   Tissue of parietal lobe of brain
Z01.4   Tissue of occipital lobe of brain
Z01.5   Tissue of cerebellum
Z01.6   Tissue of brain stem
Z01.8   Specified tissue of brain nec
Z01.9   Tissue of brain nec

Z02   **Ventricle of brain**

Z02.1   Lateral ventricle of brain
Z02.2   Third ventricle of brain
Z02.3   Fourth ventricle of brain
Z02.4   Fifth ventricle of brain
Z02.8   Specified ventricle of brain nec
Z02.9   Ventricle of brain nec

Z03   **Upper cranial nerve**

Z03.1   Olfactory nerve (i)
Z03.2   Optic nerve (ii)
Z03.3   Oculomotor nerve (iii)
Z03.4   Trochlear nerve (iv)
Z03.5   Trigeminal nerve (v)
Z03.6   Abducens nerve (vi)
Z03.8   Specified upper cranial nerve nec
Z03.9   Upper cranial nerve nec

Z04   **Other cranial nerve**

Z04.1   Facial nerve (vii)
Z04.2   Acoustic nerve (viii)
Z04.3   Glossopharyngeal nerve (ix)
Z04.4   Vagus nerve (x)
Z04.5   Accessory nerve (xi)
Z04.6   Hypoglossal nerve (xii)
Z04.7   Lower cranial nerve nec
Z04.8   Specified cranial nerve nec
Z04.9   Cranial nerve nec

Z05   **Meninges of brain**

Z05.1   Suprasellar meninges of brain
Z05.2   Meninges of middle fossa
Z05.3   Meninges of cerebellopontine angle
Z05.4   Meninges of clivus
Z05.5   Meninges of foramen magnum
Z05.6   Intraventricular meninges of brain
Z05.7   Meninges surrounding optic nerve
Z05.8   Specified meninges of brain nec
Z05.9   Meninges of brain nec

Z06 **Spinal cord**

Z06.1 Cervical spinal cord
Z06.2 Dorsal spinal cord
  Includes: Thoracic spinal cord
Z06.3 Lumbar spinal cord
Z06.4 Meninges of spinal cord
Z06.5 Cerebrospinal fluid
Z06.8 Specified spinal cord nec
Z06.9 Spinal cord nec

Z07 **Spinal nerve root**

Z07.1 Spinal nerve root of cervical spine
Z07.2 Spinal nerve root of dorsal spine
  Includes: Spinal nerve root of thoracic spine
Z07.3 Spinal nerve root of lumbar spine
Z07.8 Specified spinal nerve root nec
Z07.9 Spinal nerve root nec

Z08 **Brachial plexus**

Z08.1 Medial cord of brachial plexus
Z08.2 Lateral cord of brachial plexus
Z08.3 Posterior cord of brachial plexus
Z08.8 Specified brachial plexus nec
Z08.9 Brachial plexus nec

Z09 **Peripheral nerve of arm**

Z09.1 Circumflex nerve
Z09.2 Median nerve
Z09.3 Radial nerve
Z09.4 Ulna nerve
Z09.5 Posterior interosseous nerve
Z09.6 Anterior interosseous nerve
Z09.7 Digital nerve of finger
Z09.8 Specified peripheral nerve of arm nec
Z09.9 Peripheral nerve of arm nec

Z10 **Lumbar plexus**

Z10.1 Femoral nerve
Z10.2 Obturator nerve
Z10.3 Lateral cutaneous nerve of thigh
Z10.4 Ilioinguinal nerve
Z10.5 Iliohypogastric nerve
Z10.8 Specified lumbar plexus nec
Z10.9 Lumbar plexus nec

Z11 **Sacral plexus**

Z11.1 Sciatic nerve
Z11.2 Sacral nerve
Z11.3 Pudendal nerve
Z11.8 Specified sacral plexus nec
Z11.9 Sacral plexus nec

Z12   Other nerve

Z12.1   Popliteal nerve
Z12.2   Posterior tibial nerve
Z12.3   Sural nerve
Z12.4   Plantar nerve
Z12.5   Digital nerve of toe
Z12.6   Peripheral nerve of leg nec
Z12.7   Sympathetic nerve
Z12.8   Specified nerve nec
Z12.9   Nerve nec
        Includes: Peripheral nerve nec

Z13   Endocrine gland of neck

Z13.1   Thyroid gland
Z13.2   Aberrant thyroid tissue
Z13.3   Thyroglossal cyst
Z13.4   Thyroglossal tract
Z13.5   Parathyroid gland
Z13.8   Specified endocrine gland of neck nec
Z13.9   Endocrine gland of neck nec

Z14   Other endocrine gland

Z14.1   Pituitary gland
Z14.2   Pineal gland
Z14.3   Thymus gland
Z14.4   Adrenal gland
Z14.5   Aberrant adrenal tissue
Z14.8   Specified endocrine gland nec
Z14.9   Endocrine gland nec

Z15   Breast

Z15.1   Upper inner quadrant of breast
Z15.2   Upper outer quadrant of breast
Z15.3   Lower inner quadrant of breast
Z15.4   Lower outer quadrant of breast
Z15.5   Axillary tail of breast
Z15.6   Nipple
        Includes: Skin of nipple
Z15.8   Specified breast nec
Z15.9   Breast nec

Z16   External structure of eye

Z16.1   Orbit
Z16.2   Eyebrow
        Includes: Skin of eyebrow
Z16.3   Canthus
Z16.4   Eyelid
        Includes: Skin of eyelid
Z16.5   Lacrimal gland
Z16.6   Lacrimal sac
Z16.7   Lacrimal apparatus
Z16.8   Specified external structure of eye nec
Z16.9   External structure of eye nec

Z17　**Muscle of eye**
Includes: Tendon of muscle of eye

Z17.1　Medial rectus muscle of eye
Z17.2　Lateral rectus muscle of eye
Z17.3　Superior rectus muscle of eye
Z17.4　Inferior rectus muscle of eye
Z17.5　Superior oblique muscle of eye
Z17.6　Inferior oblique muscle of eye
Z17.7　Combinations of muscles of eye
Z17.8　Specified muscle of eye nec
Z17.9　Muscle of eye nec

Z18　**Anterior chamber of eye**

Z18.1　Conjunctiva
Z18.2　Cornea
Z18.3　Sclera
Z18.4　Iris
Z18.8　Specified anterior chamber of eye nec
Z18.9　Anterior chamber of eye nec

Z19　**Other part of eye**

Z19.1　Lens
Z19.2　Vitreous body
Z19.3　Retina
Z19.4　Choroid
Z19.8　Specified part of eye nec
Z19.9　Eye nec

Z20　**Outer ear**

Z20.1　External ear
Includes: Skin of external ear
Z20.2　External auditory canal
Z20.3　Mastoid
Includes: Attic
Z20.4　Eardrum
Z20.8　Specified outer ear nec
Z20.9　Outer ear nec

Z21　**Other part of ear**

Z21.1　Ossicle of ear
Z21.2　Middle ear
Z21.3　Eustachian canal
Z21.4　Cochlea
Z21.5　Vestibular apparatus
Z21.6　Inner ear
Z21.8　Specified part of ear nec
Z21.9　Ear nec

Z22　**Nose**

Z22.1　External nose
Includes: Skin of external nose
Z22.2　Septum of nose
Z22.3　Turbinate of nose
Z22.4　Internal nose
Z22.5　Adenoid
Z22.6　Nasopharynx
Includes: Postnasal space
Z22.8　Specified nose nec
Z22.9　Nose nec

Z23 Nasal sinus

Z23.1 Maxillary antrum
Z23.2 Frontal sinus
Z23.3 Ethmoid sinus
Z23.4 Sphenoid sinus
Z23.8 Specified nasal sinus nec
Z23.9 Nasal sinus nec

Z24 Other respiratory tract

Z24.1 Pharynx
  Excludes: Nasopharynx (Z22.6)
Z24.2 Larynx
Z24.3 Trachea
Z24.4 Carina
Z24.5 Bronchus
Z24.6 Lung
Z24.7 Mediastinum
Z24.8 Specified respiratory tract nec
Z24.9 Respiratory tract nec

Z25 Mouth

Z25.1 Lip
  Includes: Skin of lip
Z25.2 Wisdom tooth
Z25.3 Tooth nec
Z25.4 Gingiva
Z25.5 Tongue
Z25.6 Palate
Z25.7 Tonsil
  Includes: Peritonsillar region
Z25.8 Specified mouth nec
Z25.9 Mouth nec

Z26 Salivary apparatus

Z26.1 Parotid gland
Z26.2 Submandibular gland
Z26.3 Sublingual gland
Z26.4 Salivary gland
Z26.5 Parotid duct
Z26.6 Submandibular duct
Z26.7 Salivary duct
Z26.8 Specified salivary apparatus nec
Z26.9 Salivary apparatus nec

Z27 Upper digestive tract

Z27.1 Oesophagus
Z27.2 Stomach
Z27.3 Pylorus
Z27.4 Duodenum
Z27.5 Jejunum
Z27.6 Ileum
Z27.7 Small intestine
Z27.8 Specified upper digestive tract nec
Z27.9 Upper digestive tract nec

Z28   **Large intestine**

Z28.1   Appendix
Z28.2   Caecum
Z28.3   Ascending colon
Z28.4   Transverse colon
Z28.5   Descending colon
Z28.6   Sigmoid colon
Z28.7   Colon nec
Z28.8   Specified large intestine nec
Z28.9   Large intestine nec

Z29   **Other part of bowel**

Z29.1   Rectum
Z29.2   Anus
Z29.3   Perianal tissue
Z29.8   Specified part of bowel nec
Z29.9   Bowel nec

Z30   **Biliary tract**

Z30.1   Liver
Z30.2   Gall bladder
Z30.3   Common bile duct
Z30.4   Bile duct nec
         Includes: Hepatic duct
Z30.5   Sphincter of Oddi
Z30.6   Papilla of Vater
Z30.7   Ampulla of Vater
Z30.8   Specified biliary tract nec
Z30.9   Biliary tract nec

Z31   **Other abdominal organ**

Z31.1   Pancreas
Z31.2   Pancreatic duct
Z31.3   Spleen
Z31.8   Specified abdominal organ nec
Z31.9   Abdominal organ nec

Z32   **Valve of heart**

Z32.1   Mitral valve
Z32.2   Aortic valve
Z32.3   Tricuspid valve
Z32.4   Pulmonary valve
Z32.8   Specified valve of heart nec
Z32.9   Valve of heart nec

Z33   **Other part of heart**

Z33.1   Septum of atrium
Z33.2   Septum of ventricle of heart
Z33.3   Wall of heart
Z33.4   Coronary artery
Z33.5   Pericardium
Z33.8   Specified part of heart nec
Z33.9   Heart nec

Z34   Aorta

Z34.1   Ascending aorta
Z34.2   Aortic arch
Z34.3   Descending thoracic aorta
Z34.4   Thoracic aorta nec
Z34.5   Suprarenal abdominal aorta
Z34.6   Infrarenal abdominal aorta
Z34.7   Abdominal aorta nec
           Includes: Bifurcation of aorta
Z34.8   Specified aorta nec
Z34.9   Aorta nec

Z35   Cerebral artery

Z35.1   Anterior cerebral artery
Z35.2   Ophthalmic artery
Z35.3   Anterior communicating artery
Z35.4   Middle cerebral artery
Z35.5   Posterior cerebral artery
Z35.6   Posterior communicating artery
Z35.7   Artery of circle of Willis
Z35.8   Specified cerebral artery nec
Z35.9   Cerebral artery nec

Z36   Branch of thoracic aorta

Z36.1   Carotid artery
Z36.2   Subclavian artery
           Includes: Innominate artery
Z36.3   Axillary artery
Z36.4   Brachial artery
Z36.5   Vertebral artery
Z36.8   Specified branch of thoracic aorta nec
Z36.9   Branch of thoracic aorta nec

Z37   Lateral branch of abdominal aorta

Z37.1   Renal artery
Z37.2   Coeliac artery
Z37.3   Superior mesenteric artery
Z37.4   Inferior mesenteric artery
Z37.5   Suprarenal artery
Z37.8   Specified lateral branch of abdominal aorta nec
Z37.9   Lateral branch of abdominal aorta nec

Z38   Terminal branch of aorta
           Excludes: Bifurcation of aorta (Z34.7)

Z38.1   Common iliac artery
Z38.2   Internal iliac artery
Z38.3   Common femoral artery
Z38.4   Deep femoral artery
Z38.5   Superficial femoral artery
Z38.6   Popliteal artery
Z38.8   Specified terminal branch of aorta nec
Z38.9   Terminal branch of aorta nec

Z39   Vein

Z39.1   Superior vena cava
Z39.2   Inferior vena cava
Z39.3   Portal vein
Z39.4   Renal vein
Z39.5   Saphenous vein
Z39.8   Specified vein nec
Z39.9   Vein nec

Z40   Other vascular tissue

Z40.1   Pulmonary artery
Z40.2   Pulmonary vein
Z40.3   Carotid body
Z40.4   Jugular body
Z40.5   Aortic body
Z40.6   Vascular body
Z40.7   Artery nec
Z40.8   Specified vascular tissue nec
Z40.9   Vascular tissue nec

Z41   Upper urinary tract

Z41.1   Kidney
Z41.2   Ureteric orifice
           Includes: Meatus of ureter
Z41.3   Ureter nec
Z41.8   Specified upper urinary tract nec
Z41.9   Upper urinary tract nec

Z42   Lower urinary tract

Z42.1   Bladder nec
Z42.2   Prostate
Z42.3   Outlet of bladder
Z42.4   Urethral orifice
           Includes: Meatus of urethra
Z42.5   Urethra nec
Z42.6   Prepuce
           Includes: Skin of prepuce
Z42.7   Penis
           Includes: Skin of penis
Z42.8   Specified lower urinary tract nec
Z42.9   Lower urinary tract nec

Z43   Male genital organ

Z43.1   Scrotum
           Includes: Skin of scrotum
Z43.2   Testis
Z43.3   Epididymis
Z43.4   Spermatic cord
Z43.5   Seminal vesicle
Z43.6   Male perineum
           Includes: Skin of male perineum
Z43.8   Specified male genital organ nec
Z43.9   Male genital organ nec

Z44   Vagina

Z44.1   Clitoris
Z44.2   Bartholin gland
            Includes: Bartholin duct
Z44.3   Vulva
            Includes: Skin of vulva
Z44.4   Female perineum
            Includes: Skin of female perineum
Z44.5   Introitus of vagina
Z44.6   Pouch of Douglas
Z44.8   Specified vagina nec
Z44.9   Vagina nec

Z45   Uterus

Z45.1   Cervix uteri
Z45.2   Gravid uterus
            Includes: Delivered uterus
Z45.3   Fetus
Z45.4   Placenta
Z45.5   Amniotic membrane
Z45.8   Specified uterus nec
Z45.9   Uterus nec

Z46   Other female genital tract

Z46.1   Fimbria
Z46.2   Fallopian tube
Z46.3   Ovary
Z46.4   Broad ligament of uterus
Z46.8   Specified female genital tract nec
Z46.9   Female genital tract nec

Z47   Skin of face
            Includes: Sebcutaneous tissue of face
            Excludes: Eyebrow (Z16.2)
                        Skin of eyelid (Z16.4)
                        Skin of external ear (Z20.1)
                        Skin of external nose (Z22.1)
                        Lip (Z25.1)

Z47.1   Skin of forehead
Z47.2   Skin of temple
Z47.3   Skin of cheek
Z47.4   Skin of nasolabial area
Z47.5   Skin of chin
Z47.8   Specified skin of face nec
Z47.9   Skin of face nec

Z48   Skin of other part of head or neck
            Includes: Subcutaneous tissue of other part of head or neck

Z48.1   Skin of scalp
Z48.2   Skin of neck
Z48.8   Skin of specified part of head nec
Z48.9   Skin of head nec

Z49   **Skin of trunk**
         Includes: Subcutaneous tissue of trunk
         Excludes: Skin of prepuce (Z42.6)
                 Skin of penis (Z42.7)
                 Skin of scrotum (Z43.1)
                 Skin of male perineum (Z43.6)
                 Skin of vulva (Z44.3)
                 Skin of female perineum (Z44.4)

Z49.1   Skin of breast
         Excludes: Nipple (Z15.6)
Z49.2   Skin of axilla
Z49.3   Skin of anterior trunk
Z49.4   Skin of back
Z49.5   Skin of buttock
Z49.8   Specified skin of trunk nec
Z49.9   Skin of trunk nec

Z50   **Skin of other site**
         Includes: Subcutaneous tissue of other site

Z50.1   Skin of arm
Z50.2   Skin of hand
Z50.3   Skin of finger
Z50.4   Skin of leg
Z50.5   Skin of foot
Z50.6   Skin of toe
Z50.8   Skin of specified site nec
Z50.9   Skin nec

Z51   **Nail**

Z51.1   Nail bed
Z51.8   Specified nail nec
Z51.9   Nail nec

Z52   **Chest wall**

Z52.1   Pleura
Z52.2   Pleural cavity
Z52.8   Specified chest wall nec
Z52.9   Chest wall nec

Z53   **Abdominal wall**

Z53.1   Diaphragm
Z53.2   Umbilicus
         Includes: Skin of umbilicus
Z53.3   Peritoneum
Z53.4   Peritoneal cavity
Z53.5   Omentum
Z53.6   Mesentery
Z53.8   Specified abdominal wall nec
Z53.9   Abdominal wall nec

Z54   **Muscle of shoulder or upper arm**
         Includes: Tendon of muscle of shoulder or upper arm

Z54.1   Deltoid
Z54.2   Rotator cuff of shoulder
Z54.3   Pectoralis
Z54.4   Biceps brachii
         Includes: Brachial muscle nec
Z54.5   Triceps brachii
Z54.8   Specified muscle of shoulder or upper arm nec
Z54.9   Muscle of shoulder or upper arm nec

Z55   **Muscle of forearm**
Includes: Tendon of muscle of forearm

Z55.1   Flexor muscle of forearm
Z55.2   Extensor muscle of forearm
Z55.3   Supinator muscle of forearm
Z55.4   Pronator muscle of forearm
Z55.5   Palmaris longus
Z55.8   Specified muscle of forearm nec
Z55.9   Muscle of forearm nec

Z56   **Muscle of hand**
Includes: Tendon of muscle of hand

Z56.1   Flexor pollicis longus
Z56.2   Thenar muscle
Z56.3   Flexor digitorum superficialis
Z56.4   Flexor digitorum profundus
Z56.5   Hypothenar muscle
Z56.6   Interosseous muscle of hand
        Includes: Lumbrical muscle of hand
Z56.7   Extensor muscle of hand
Z56.8   Specified muscle of hand nec
Z56.9   Muscle of hand nec

Z57   **Muscle of hip or thigh**
Includes: Tendon of muscle of hip or thigh

Z57.1   Gluteus
        Includes: Short hip rotator muscle
Z57.2   Iliopsoas
Z57.3   Quadriceps
Z57.4   Adductor muscle of thigh
        Includes: Adductor muscle of hip
Z57.5   Tensor fasciae latae
Z57.6   Biceps femoris
Z57.7   Hamstring
Z57.8   Specified muscle of hip or thigh nec
Z57.9   Muscle of hip or thigh nec

Z58   **Muscle of lower leg**
Includes: Tendon of lower leg

Z58.1   Triceps surae
        Includes: Tendo achillis
Z58.2   Peroneus
Z58.3   Tibialis posterior
Z58.4   Tibialis anterior
Z58.5   Extensor hallucis longus
Z58.6   Extensor digitorum muscle of foot
Z58.7   Infrapatellar tendon
Z58.8   Specified muscle of lower leg nec
Z58.9   Muscle of lower leg nec

Z59   **Muscle of foot**
Includes: Tendon of muscle of foot

Z59.1   Flexor hallucis longus
Z59.2   Flexor digitorum muscle of foot
Z59.3   Short hallux muscle
Z59.4   Short sole muscle
Z59.5   Interosseous muscle of foot
Z59.6   Lumbrical muscle of foot
Z59.8   Specified muscle of foot nec
Z59.9   Muscle of foot nec

Z60 **Other muscle**
Includes: Tendon of muscle nec

Z60.1 Muscle of face
Z60.2 Muscle of neck
Z60.3 Muscle of anterior abdominal wall
Z60.4 Muscle of back
Z60.8 Specified muscle nec
Z60.9 Muscle nec

Z61 **Lymph node**

Z61.1 Cervical lymph node
Z61.2 Scalene lymph node
Z61.3 Axillary lymph node
Z61.4 Mediastinal lymph node
Z61.5 Paraaortic lymph node
Z61.6 Inguinal lymph node
Z61.8 Specified lymph node nec
Z61.9 Lymph node nec

Z62 **Other soft tissue**

Z62.1 Fascia
Z62.2 Lymphatic duct
Z62.3 Lymphatic tissue
Z62.4 Connective tissue
Z62.8 Specified soft tissue nec
Z62.9 Soft tissue nec

Z63 **Bone of cranium**

Z63.1 Frontal bone
Z63.2 Parietal bone
Z63.3 Temporal bone
Z63.4 Occipital bone
Z63.8 Specified bone of cranium nec
Z63.9 Bone of cranium nec

Z64 **Bone of face**

Z64.1 Nasoethmoid complex of bones
Z64.2 Nasal bone
Z64.3 Zygomatic complex of bones
Z64.4 Maxilla
Z64.8 Specified bone of face nec
Z64.9 Bone of face nec

Z65 **Jaw**

Z65.1 Mandible
Z65.2 Temporomandibular joint
Z65.8 Specified jaw nec
Z65.9 Jaw nec

Z66 **Vertebra**

Z66.1 Atlas
Z66.2 Axis bone
Z66.3 Cervical vertebra
Z66.4 Thoracic vertebra
Z66.5 Lumbar vertebra
Z66.8 Specified vertebra nec
Z66.9 Vertebra nec

Z67   **Intervertebral joint**

Z67.1   Atlantooccipital joint
Z67.2   Atlantoaxial joint
Z67.3   Cervical intervertebral joint
Z67.4   Thoracic intervertebral joint
Z67.5   Lumbar intervertebral joint
Z67.6   Lumbosacral joint
Z67.8   Specified intervertebral joint nec
Z67.9   Intervertebral joint nec

Z68   **Bone of shoulder girdle**

Z68.1   Clavicle
Z68.2   Acromion process of scapula
Z68.3   Coracoid process of scapula
Z68.4   Glenoid cavity of scapula
Z68.5   Scapula nec
Z68.8   Specified bone of shoulder girdle nec
Z68.9   Bone of shoulder girdle nec

Z69   **Humerus**

Z69.1   Head of humerus
Z69.2   Tuberosity of humerus
Z69.3   Neck of humerus
Z69.4   Mid shaft of humerus
Z69.5   Lateral condyle of humerus
Z69.6   Medial epicondyle of humerus
Z69.7   Lower end of humerus nec
       Includes: Articular surface of humerus at elbow
Z69.8   Specified humerus nec
Z69.9   Humerus nec

Z70   **Radius**

Z70.1   Head of radius
Z70.2   Neck of radius
Z70.3   Shaft of radius nec
Z70.4   Styloid process of radius
Z70.5   Lower end of radius nec
       Includes: Articular surface of radius at wrist
Z70.8   Specified radius nec
Z70.9   Radius nec

Z71   **Ulna**

Z71.1   Olecranon process of ulna
Z71.2   Shaft of ulna nec
Z71.3   Coronoid process of ulna
Z71.4   Head of ulna
       Includes: Articular surface of ulna at elbow
Z71.5   Styloid process of ulna
Z71.6   Lower end of ulna nec
Z71.8   Specified ulna nec
Z71.9   Ulna nec

Z72   **Other bone of arm or wrist**

Z72.1   Shafts of radius and ulna in combination
Z72.2   Scaphoid bone
Z72.3   Lunate
Z72.4   Carpal bone
       Includes: Articular surface of carpus at wrist
Z72.8   Specified bone of arm or wrist nec
Z72.9   Bone of arm or wrist nec

Z73   **Other bone of hand**

Z73.1   First metacarpal
Z73.2   Metacarpal nec
Z73.3   Phalanx of thumb
Z73.4   Phalanx of finger
Z73.8   Specified bone of hand nec
Z73.9   Bone of hand nec

Z74   **Rib cage**

Z74.1   Manubrium sterni
Z74.2   Sternum nec
Z74.3   First rib
Z74.4   Second to tenth rib
Z74.5   Eleventh or twelfth rib
Z74.6   Rib nec
Z74.8   Specified rib cage nec
Z74.9   Rib cage nec

Z75   **Bone of pelvis**

Z75.1   Body of sacrum
Z75.2   Ala of sacrum
Z75.3   Wing of ilium
Z75.4   Ischium
Z75.5   Ramus of pubis
Z75.6   Acetabulum
Z75.7   Coccyx
Z75.8   Specified bone of pelvis nec
Z75.9   Bone of pelvis nec

Z76   **Femur**

Z76.1   Head of femur
Z76.2   Neck of femur
Z76.3   Trochanter of femur
Z76.4   Shaft of femur
Z76.5   Lower end of femur nec
        Includes: Articular surface of femur at knee
Z76.8   Specified femur nec
Z76.9   Femur nec

Z77   **Tibia**

Z77.1   Condyle of tibia
Z77.2   Shaft of tibia nec
Z77.3   Medial malleolus
Z77.4   Upper end of tibia nec
        Includes: Articular surface of tibia at knee
Z77.5   Lower end of tibia nec
        Includes: Articular surface of tibia at ankle
Z77.8   Specified tibia nec
Z77.9   Tibia nec

Z78   **Other bone of lower leg**

Z78.1   Shafts of tibia and fibula in combination
Z78.2   Head of fibula
Z78.3   Shaft of fibula nec
Z78.4   Lateral malleolus
Z78.5   Lower end of fibula nec
        Includes: Articular surface of fibula at ankle
Z78.6   Fibula nec
Z78.7   Patella
Z78.8   Specified bone of lower leg nec
Z78.9   Bone of lower leg nec

Z79 Bone of tarsus

Z79.1 Talus
Includes: Articular surface of talus at ankle
Z79.2 Os calcis
Z79.3 Navicular bone of foot
Z79.4 Cuboid bone
Z79.5 Cuneiform bone
Z79.8 Specified bone of tarsus nec
Z79.9 Bone of tarsus nec

Z80 Other bone of foot

Z80.1 First metatarsal
Z80.2 Metatarsal nec
Z80.3 Phalanx of great toe
Z80.4 Phalanx of toe nec
Z80.8 Specified bone of foot nec
Z80.9 Bone of foot nec

Z81 Joint of shoulder girdle or arm
Note: For operations on one bone of joint use site code for bone in preference to site code for joint (Z68-Z80)

Z81.1 Sternoclavicular joint
Z81.2 Acromioclavicular joint
Z81.3 Glenohumeral joint
Z81.4 Shoulder joint
Z81.5 Elbow joint
Z81.6 Superior radioulnar joint
Z81.7 Inferior radioulnar joint
Z81.8 Specified joint of shoulder girdle or arm nec
Z81.9 Joint of shoulder girdle or arm nec

Z82 Joint of wrist or hand
Note at Z81 applies

Z82.1 Radiocarpal joint
Z82.2 Intercarpal joint
Z82.3 Carpometacarpal joint of thumb
Z82.4 Carpometacarpal joint of finger
Z82.8 Specified joint of wrist or hand nec
Z82.9 Joint of wrist or hand nec

Z83 Joint of finger
Note at Z81 applies

Z83.1 Metacarpophalangeal joint of thumb
Z83.2 Metacarpophalangeal joint of finger
Z83.3 Interphalangeal joint of thumb
Z83.4 Proximal interphalangeal joint of finger
Z83.5 Distal interphalangeal joint of finger
Z83.6 Interphalangeal joint of finger nec
Z83.8 Specified joint of finger nec
Z83.9 Joint of finger nec

Z84 Joint of pelvis or upper leg
Note at Z81 applies

Z84.1 Sacroiliac joint
Z84.2 Pubic symphysis
Z84.3 Hip joint
Z84.4 Patellofemoral joint
Z84.5 Tibiofemoral joint
Z84.6 Knee joint
Z84.8 Specified joint of pelvis or upper leg nec
Z84.9 Joint of pelvis or upper leg nec

Z85   **Joint of lower leg or tarsus**
Note at Z81 applies

Z85.1   Upper tibiofibular joint
Z85.2   Lower tibiofibular joint
Z85.3   Talocalcaneal joint
Z85.4   Talonavicular joint
Z85.5   Calcaneocuboid joint
Z85.6   Ankle joint
Z85.8   Specified joint of lower leg or tarsus nec
Z85.9   Joint of lower leg or tarsus nec

Z86   **Other joint of foot**
Note at Z81 applies

Z86.1   Mid tarsal joint
Z86.2   Intertarsal joint
Z86.3   Tarsometatarsal joint
Z86.4   Metatarsophalangeal joint of great toe
Z86.5   Metatarsophalangeal joint of toe nec
Z86.6   Interphalangeal joint of toe
Z86.8   Specified joint of foot nec
Z86.9   Joint of foot nec

Z87   **Other part of musculoskeletal system**

Z87.1   Bone nec
Z87.2   Ligament of joint
Z87.3   Capsule of joint
Z87.4   Joint nec
Z87.8   Specified part of musculoskeletal system nec
Z87.9   Musculoskeletal system nec

Z89   **Arm region**
Note: *These codes should not normally be used when more specific site codes may be identified (Z01-Z87)*

Z89.1   Shoulder nec
Z89.2   Upper arm nec
Z89.3   Forearm nec
Z89.4   Hand nec
Z89.5   Thumb nec
Z89.6   Finger nec
Z89.8   Specified arm region nec
Z89.9   Arm nec

Z90   **Leg region**
Note at Z89 applies

Z90.1   Buttock nec
Z90.2   Hip nec
Z90.3   Upper leg nec
Z90.4   Lower leg nec
Z90.5   Foot nec
Z90.6   Great toe nec
Z90.7   Toe nec
Z90.8   Specified leg region nec
Z90.9   Leg nec

Z92   Other region of body
Note at Z89 applies

Z92.1   Head nec
Z92.2   Face nec
Z92.3   Neck nec
Z92.4   Chest nec
Z92.5   Back nec
Z92.6   Abdomen nec
Z92.7   Trunk nec
Z92.8   Specified region of body nec
Z92.9   Region of body nec

Z94   Laterality of operation

Z94.1   Bilateral operation
Z94.2   Right sided operation
Z94.3   Left sided operation
Z94.4   Unilateral operation
Z94.8   Specified laterality nec
Z94.9   Laterality nec

Printed in the United Kingdom for HMSO
Dd 292762   C8   6/90